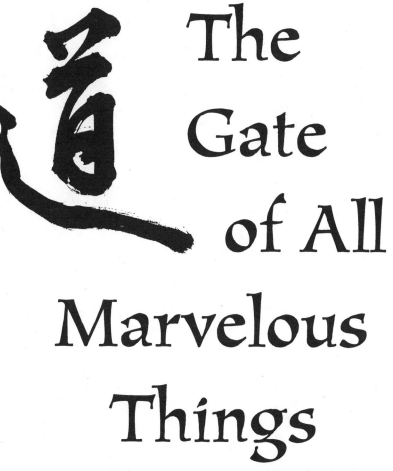

The Gate of All Marvelous Things

A Guide to Reading the Tao Te Ching

Translated by Gregory C. Richter

Red Mansions Publishing
South San Francisco, California

Cover design by Linda Revel
Text design by Wendy K. Lee
This book was typeset using the Apple Language Kit. Additonal characters designed by Wendy K. Lee.

First Edition 1998
Printed in Canada

ISBN: 1-891688-00-6
Library of Congress Catalog Card Number: 98-65306

Distributed by
China Books and Periodicals, Inc.
2929 24th Street
San Francisco CA 94110
www.chinabooks.com

Table of Contents

Introduction

More and more students of Chinese are becoming familiar with the *pinyin* transcription system; instructional materials in *pinyin* enable students to build on their knowledge of the language before they have mastered Chinese characters. Unique in conception and format, this new translation of *Dào Dé Jīng* (Tao Te Ching) by Lǎozǐ (Lao Tzu) is the first to feature a *pinyin* transcription of the Chinese text; the transcription indicates current standard Mandarin pronunciation (which, of course is not the pronunciation used by Lǎozǐ in the fifth century B.C.!) Not a scholarly commentary, the volume is designed especially for students of Chinese seeking an introduction to *Dào Dé Jīng*. The *pinyin* text is accompanied not only by an English translation, but also by a word for word gloss. The volume will also be of use to readers without knowledge of Chinese seeking a detailed, usable translation; all readers will gain a feeling for the extreme succinctness of Classical Chinese — and for the difficulties facing the translator.

In this edition, the Chinese characters *(hànzì)* reflect the text in simplified characters as it appears in **_Dào Dé Jīng_** 道德经 1990 Anhui People's Publishing Co. Annotated in Chinese by Xú Shù and Liú Háo. For line divisions and punctuation of the Chinese text, I have followed my own preferences. The *pinyin* transcription of the text always appears on the second line. In the *pinyin* transcription, I have not generally taken tone adjustment rules into consideration, e.g. I write *kěyǐ* "CAN" rather than *kéyǐ,* but before falling tone I transcribe *bù* "NOT" as *bú*, e.g. *bú hài* "NOT HARM."

The gloss, always on the third line, is a word for word translation of the Chinese text. All items in the gloss are capitalized. The translation, on the fourth line, renders the meaning in normal English; often, it is necessary to provide paraphrases for words in the gloss. In the translation, those words directly carried over from the gloss retain their capitalization; paraphrases shorter than the corresponding gloss or of equal length also maintain their capitalization, e.g. *lì qì* is glossed "SHARP IMPLEMENT" but translated as "WEAPON;" *qiáng* is glossed "STRONGLY" but translated in context as "RESOLUTELY." Other English words in the translation — those which must be inserted to create complete sentences or to clarify the meaning —appear in lower case, e.g. in No. 19, *wú yōu* is glossed as "NOT WORRY" but translated "and there will be NO WORRY." (When interpolated, the pronoun "I" and initial article "A" are indicated in small capitals.) In general, verbs in the gloss are uninflected and nouns in the gloss show no number; normal endings appear in the translation. Given these conventions, readers can easily see how much of the translation directly reflects the Chinese text, and how much is interpolated. For idioms, a strictly etymological gloss seemed helpful. Thus, *bǎi xìng* is glossed as "HUNDRED SURNAME," but translated as "PEOPLE." Sometimes, though, the gloss indicates not a literal translation, but only the equivalent English word in context, e.g. *yī guān* in No. 1 is glossed (and translated) "TO OBSERVE," though a more literal version might be "TAKE OBSERVE." Throughout, I have attempted to keep unnecessary interpretation to a minimum. In some cases, though, the urge to interpret proved irresistible. Thus, faced with two apparent riddles in No. 9, I have supplied "VESSEL" and "KNIFE" though these correspond only to *zhī* in the Chinese text ("IT" in the gloss).

Lacking consistent English equivalents, Chinese grammatical particles are often glossed simply as [PART]. This seemed more appropriate than developing a complex set of abbreviations reflecting a complex morphological analysis. The translation should help to clarify the function of a given particle in context; typically, a given particle can be utilized in a range of functions. The particle *zhī*, for example, sometimes serves as a direct object pronoun; elsewhere it may serve to mark a possessor or a modifier, though it is sometimes difficult to differentiate these two functions. For direct object function, I employ glosses such as "HIM" or "IT," but otherwise I gloss *zhī* as [PART]. The particle *qí* also deserves special comment; it, too, is employed in a range of functions. When its technical function is that of possessive marker, I have chosen English renderings such as "ONE'S" or "ITS," but it should be kept in mind that there is sometimes no antecedent. That is, this particle may indicate that an entity merely belongs to "someone" — or the reference may simply be to the entity in general. Thus, in No. 4, *tóng qí chén* is glossed as "UNITE ITS DUST," but translated simply as "... UNITES with

DUST." This usage is characteristic not only of Lǎozǐ, but also of Zhuāngzǐ and other authors writing in Classical Chinese.

Surprisingly often, word order in Chinese and English coincides. In other cases, of course, English syntax differs from that of Chinese. Thus, *tiān xià*, glossed as "HEAVEN UNDER," can be translated as "UNDER HEAVEN" or "all things UNDER HEAVEN." (In other cases, this term is translated as "UNIVERSE"). Sometimes a translated item may be physically far removed from the corresponding gloss, but the correspondence should become apparent if one analyzes both lines carefully. Occasionally, two *hànzì* appear above an English gloss: they are treated as an unanalyzed two-character compound — a single word with a single gloss. Thus, for *míngbái*, in lieu of providing the irrelevant etymological analysis "BRIGHT WHITE," the gloss appears simply as "UNDERSTAND." When two transcriptions are linked with a hyphen, the compound is analyzed: each component receives a separate gloss, but the entire compound corresponds to a single word on the translation line, e.g. *qīng-jìng*, glossed as "CLEAR-CALM" and translated "TRANQUILITY." (Two-character compounds are far less common in Lǎozǐ's writing than they are in Modern Chinese.) A hyphen linking two or more words in the gloss may indicate that the entire unit corresponds to a single *hànzì*, e.g. *gōng* is glossed as "MERITORIOUS-ACT."

Throughout, since the term is well established in English, *dào* —literally "ROAD" or "WAY" — is glossed and translated as "DAO" when used in the metaphysical sense. I employ the spelling "DAO" (rather than "TAO") to reflect the conventions of *pinyin*. Similarly, *yīn* appears in English as "YIN" and *yáng* is rendered as "YANG". For other key philosophical terms, I have selected native English equivalents: *dé* is glossed and translated throughout as "VIRTUE," *cí* as "KINDNESS," *rén* as "BENEVOLENCE," *yì* as "RIGHTEOUSNESS," *lǐ* as "RITE" or "RITUAL," and *qì* as "FORCE" or "INNER FORCE." *Shàn* is more challenging, but is variously translated as "GOOD," "WELL," "KIND," or "ADEPT." *Wàn wù*, glossed "TEN-THOUSAND THING," is generally translated "ALL THINGS" as this is apparently the sense intended. The title of the work is not translated, but for *Dào Dé Jīng* one might propose the gloss "WAY VIRTUE CLASSIC;" a reasonable translation might be "BOOK of the WAY and of VIRTUE."

It must be kept in mind that *Dào Dé Jīng* is a highly ambiguous text: in many cases, multiple possibilities present themselves. Sometimes it is difficult to make a choice; in the Chinese text, a single word may convey several semantic values simultaneously. In No. 55, for example, *míng* brings to mind not only the brightness of light, but also intelligence and enlightenment. I have chosen the translation "BRIGHTNESS," but it is difficult to find an English term which clearly conveys all the connotations of the Chinese one. Indeed, one often has the feeling that Lǎozǐ was playing with the text — that he took delight in writing ambiguously — but in an unannotated translation such as this, it is generally necessary to choose one solution only. Occasionally, though, one can have it both ways. No. 53, for example, contains a play on words: here, *dào* means both "ROAD" and "DAO," so I have adopted the translation "ROAD of the dao." In some cases context does assist in determining shades of meaning: in various contexts, the same word (Chinese character) may receive many different glosses and translations. Thus l̀ì means either "SHARP" or "BENEFIT." In the context of weapons (No. 36), "SHARP" is the likely choice, but in describing the dao, *lì ér bú hài* in No. 81 is translated "BENEFITS AND does NOT HARM." Elsewhere, though, it is <u>not</u> the various senses of a single word that are at issue. Rather, Chinese contains many distinct but homophonous words written with distinct characters, e.g. *dào* "DAO" and *dào* "BANDIT;" *mǔ* "MOTHER" and *mǔ* "MASCULINE;" *míng* "BRIGHT," *míng* "DARK," and *míng* "NAME." To determine whether one is dealing with various senses of a single word, or with translations of distinct but homophonous words, one must compare the corresponding characters in the *hànzì* text.

Unavoidably, some renderings in the current translation are influenced by annotations and translations appearing in other editions of *Dào Dé Jīng*; this extends to the resolution of the ambiguities as well. In No. 1, for example, *wú míng* is ambiguous: *wú míng tiān dì zhī shǐ* could be translated "NOTH-INGNESS is the NAME of the BEGINNING of HEAVEN AND EARTH" or simply "The NAME-LESS is the BEGINNING OF HEAVEN AND EARTH." Given the subsequent discussions of *wú* as a metaphysical concept in its own right, e.g. in Nos. 1 and 40, I have chosen — with Xú and Liú — to adopt the first possibility. Admittedly, though, there are arguments for the second translation as well. Thus, in Nos. 32 and 37, *wú míng* clearly means "NAMELESS."

To the extent possible, I have translated in a non-sexist manner. This is facilitated by the very ambiguity of the text: grammatical number can often be taken as plural, obviating the need to select a gender. Thus, in No. 33 one might propose the translation "He who does NOT LOSE what HE POS-SESSES," but I have instead chosen the plural: "Those who do NOT LOSE what THEY POSSESS." References to "the SAGE," however, are taken as masculine singular.

This book makes no claim to be definitive; it is only one of many possibilities. Still, having read this version of the text, students wishing to delve into the "meaning behind the meaning" will be better prepared to conduct further research. Some English translations may sound more "poetic," but lyricism comes at a cost. Many translations stray widely from the text, romanticizing it or omitting content, but I have chosen to be more rigorous in making the English and Chinese texts correspond. Though this translation is certainly not the most lyrical one, it strives to be a clear and accessible one, enhancing its value for readers seeking to gain basic familiarity with *Dào Dé Jīng*.

Thanks to David Wakefield for many interesting conversations on the *Dào Dé Jīng*.

Special thanks to Jiang Yizhu for inputting the Chinese characters, and for her very helpful com-ments on the book.

A *Pinyin* Pronunciation Guide

Pinyin transcriptions are generally easy to interpret. The pronunciation of most letters is very similar to the English pronunciation. The exceptions are listed below. Here again, the pronunciations are very similar to the English sounds listed, but in order to develop a good accent it is essential to listen to native speakers of Chinese.

CONSONANTS

c = English **ts**

g = English **g** as in **go** (always)

q = English **ch**

r (beginning of Chinese word) = American English **s** as in **vision**   + American English **r** — simultaneously.

r (end of Chinese word) = American English **r**

x = English **sh**

z = English **dz**

zh = English **j**

VOWELS

e = English **u** as in **up**
    BUT **ye** = English **ye** as in **yes**

i = English **i** as in **machine**
    BUT **chi** = **chr** (Rhymes with English **her**.)
      shi = **shr** (Rhymes with English **her**.)
      zhi = **zhr** (Rhymes with English **her**.)
      ri = long Chinese **r**
      ci = **ts** + English **oo** as in **took**, but with lips drawn back
      si = **ts** + English **oo** as in **took**, but with lips drawn back
      zi = **dz** + English **oo** as in **took**, but with lips drawn back

o (not before **ng**) = English **o** as in **or**

    BUT **bo** = **bwo** (with **o** as in English **or**)
      po = **pwo** (with **o** as in English **or**)
      mo = **mwo** (with **o** as in English **or**)
      fo = **fwo** (with **o** as in English **or**)

o (before **ng**) = English **u** as in **rude**

ü = English **i** as in **machine**, but with lips rounded

u (not before **n**) = English **u** as in **rude**

   BUT **ju = jü**
        qu = chü
        xu = shü
        yu = yü

u (before **n**) = English **wo** as in **woman**

   BUT **jun = jün**
        qun = chün
        xun = shün
        yun = yün

a (not before **n**) = English **a** as in **father**

a (before **n**) = English **a** as in **fat**

   BUT **-ian** = English **yen**
        yan = English **yen**
        juan = jü + English **en** as in **yen**
        quan = chü + English **en** as in **yen**
        xuan = shü + English **en** as in **yen**
        yuan = yü + English **en** as in **yen**

DIPHTHONGS and TRIPHTHONGS

These are sequences of two or three vowels, e.g. **ia, iao, ue**.
The components are pronounced in sequence to form the nucleus of a single syllable. Pronunciation is generally predictable from the basic values of the vowels; some exceptions have already been listed above when relevant. Remaining exceptions are as follows:

ue = ü + English **e** as in **yes**

ie = English **ye** as in **yes**

ei = English **é** as in **fiancé**

iu = y + American English **o** as in **owe**

ou = American English **o** as in **owe**

ui = American English **way**

TONES

Chinese has four tones. Generally, each syllable has a tone, but occasionally a syllable may occur without tone. The transcription of the four tones can be illustrated with the vowel **a**.

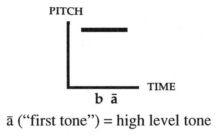

ā ("first tone") = high level tone

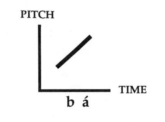

á ("second tone") = rising tone

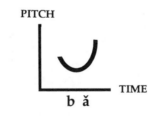

ǎ ("third tone") = falling rising tone (slight fall + sharp rise)

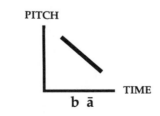

à ("fourth tone") = falling tone

Chapter 1

道　可　道，非　常　道。
dào　kě　dào,　fēi　cháng　dào.
DAO　CAN　EXPLAIN,　NOT　UNCHANGING　DAO.
The DAO which one CAN EXPLAIN is NOT the UNCHANGING DAO.

名　可　名，非　常　名。
míng　kě　míng　fēi　cháng　míng.
NAME　CAN　NAME　NOT　UNCHANGING　NAME.
The NAME which one CAN NAME is NOT the UNCHANGING NAME.

无，名　天　地　之　始。
wú,　míng　tiān　dì　zhī　shǐ.
NOTHINGNESS, NAME　HEAVEN　EARTH　[PART]　BEGINNING.
NOTHINGNESS is the NAME of the BEGINNING OF HEAVEN and EARTH.

有，名　万　物　之　母。
yǒu,　míng　wàn　wù　zhī　mǔ.
EXISTENCE,　NAME　TEN-THOUSAND　THING　[PART]　MOTHER.
EXISTENCE is the NAME of the MOTHER OF ALL THINGS.

故　常　无，
gù　cháng　wú,
THEREFORE　ALWAYS　NOTHINGNESS,
THEREFORE one should ALWAYS emphasize NOTHINGNESS

欲　以　观　其　妙；
yù　yǐ　guān　qí　miào;
DESIRE　TO　OBSERVE　ITS　MARVELOUSNESS;
If one DESIRES TO OBSERVE the MARVELOUSNESS of the dao;

常　　有，　欲　　以　　观　　其　　徼。

cháng　　yǒu,　　yù　　yǐ　　guān　　qí　　jiào.

ALWAYS　EXISTENCE,　DESIRE　TO　OBSERVE　ITS　LIMIT.

One should ALWAYS emphasize EXISTENCE if one DESIRES TO OBSERVE the LIMITS of the dao.

此　　两　　者，　同　　出　　而　　异　　名；

cǐ　　liáng　　zhě,　　tóng　　chū　　ér　　yì　　míng;

THESE　TWO　[PART],　SAME　ORIGIN　BUT　DIFFERENT　NAME;

THESE TWO have the SAME ORIGIN BUT DIFFERENT NAMES;

同　　谓　　之　　玄。

tóng　　wèi　　zhī　　xuán.

BOTH　CALL　THEM　PROFOUND.

One can CALL BOTH of THEM PROFOUND.

玄　　之　　又　　玄，

xuán　　zhī　　yòu　　xuán,

PROFOUND　[PART]　MORE　PROFOUND,

MORE PROFOUND than PROFOUND,

众　　妙　　之　　门。

zhòng　　miào　　zhī　　mén.

ALL　MARVELOUS　[PART]　GATE.

They are the GATE OF ALL MARVELOUS things.

天　下　皆　知　美　之　为　美，

tiān　xià　jiē　zhī　měi　zhī　wéi　měi,

HEAVEN　UNDER　ALL　KNOW　BEAUTIFUL　[PART]　BE　BEAUTIFUL,

UNDER HEAVEN EVERYONE KNOWS** that the capacity **OF** the **BEAUTIFUL** to **BE BEAUTIFUL

斯　恶　矣;

sī　è　yǐ;

DEPEND　UGLY　[PART];

DEPENDS** on the existence of the **UGLY;

皆　知　善　之　为　善，

jiē　zhī　shàn　zhī　wéi　shàn,

ALL　KNOW　KIND　[PART]　BE　KIND,

EVERYONE KNOWS** that the capacity **OF KINDNESS** to **BE KIND

斯　不　善　矣。

sī　bú　shàn　yǐ.

DEPEND　NOT　KIND　[PART].

DEPENDS** on the existence of the **UNKIND.

有　无　相　生，

yǒu　wú　xiāng　shēng,

EXISTENCE　NOTHINGNESS　MUTUALLY　BORN,

EXISTENCE** and **NOTHINGNESS** are **MUTUALLY BORN,

难　易　相　成，

nán　yì　xiāng　chéng,

DIFFICULT　EASY　MUTUALLY　COMPLEMENT,

***DIFFICULT** and **EASY MUTUALLY COMPLEMENT** one another,*

长　　短　　相　　形，

cháng　　*duǎn*　　*xiāng*　　*xíng,*
LONG　　SHORT　　MUTUALLY　　SHAPE,

LONG and SHORT MUTUALLY SHAPE one another,

高　　下　　相　　盈，

gāo　　*xià*　　*xiāng*　　*yíng,*
TALL　　SHORT　　MUTUALLY　　FILL,

TALL and SHORT MUTUALLY FILL one another,

音　　声　　相　　和，

yīn　　*shēng*　　*xiāng*　　*hé,*
SOUND　　MUSIC　　MUTUALLY　　HARMONIZE,

SOUND and MUSIC MUTUALLY HARMONIZE,

前　　后　　相　　随；

qián　　*hòu*　　*xiāng*　　*suí;*
BEFORE　　AFTER　　MUTUALLY　　FOLLOW;

BEFORE and AFTER MUTUALLY FOLLOW one another;

恒　　也。

héng　　*yě.*
BALANCE　　[PART].

There is BALANCE.

是　以　圣　人　处　无　为　之　事。

shì　*yǐ*　*shèng-*　*rén*　*chǔ*　*wú*　*wéi*　*zhī*　*shì.*
BE　WHY　SAGACIOUS-　PERSON　ENGAGE　NOT　ACT　[PART]　AFFAIR.

This IS WHY the SAGE ENGAGES in NON-ACTION.

行　不　言　之　教。
xíng　bù　yán　zhī　jiào.
ENGAGE　NOT　SPEAK　[PART]　TEACH.

He ENGAGES in TEACHING by NOT SPEAKING.

万　物　作　而　弗　始。
wàn　wù　zuò　ér　fú　shǐ.
TEN-THOUSAND　THING　ACHIEVE　BUT　NOT　UNDERTAKE.

He ACHIEVES ALL THINGS BUT UNDERTAKES NOTHING.

生　而　弗　有。
shēng　ér　fú　yǒu.
PRODUCE　BUT　NOT　HAVE.

He PRODUCES BUT HAS NOTHING.

为　而　不　恃。
wéi　ér　bú　shì.
ACT　BUT　NOT　DEPEND.

He ACTS BUT does NOT DEPEND.

功　成　而　弗　居。
gōng　chéng　ér　fú　jū.
MERITORIOUS-ACT　ACCOMPLISH　BUT　NOT　POSSESS.

He ACCOMPLISHES MERITORIOUS ACTS BUT does NOT POSSESS.

夫　唯　弗　居，是　以　不　去。
fú　wéi　fú　jū,　shì　yǐ　bú　qù.
SINCE　NOT　POSSESS,　BE　WHY　NOT　LOST.

SINCE he does NOT POSSESS he is NOT LOST.

5

Chapter 3

不　尚　贤，使　民　不　争。
bú　shàng　xián,　shǐ　mín　bù　zhēng.
NOT　REWARD　CAPABLE,　CAUSE　PEOPLE　NOT　CONTEND.

NOT REWARDING the CAPABLE ENSURES that the PEOPLE will NOT CONTEND.

不　贵　难　得　之　货，
bú　guì　nán　dé　zhī　huò,
NOT　VALUE　DIFFICULT　OBTAIN　[PART]　COMMODITY,

NOT VALUING RARE COMMODITIES

使　民　不　为　盗。
shǐ　mín　bù　wéi　dào.
CAUSE　PEOPLE　NOT　PRACTICE　THIEVERY.

ENSURES that the PEOPLE will NOT PRACTICE THIEVERY.

不　见　可　欲，使　民　心　不　乱。
bú　jiàn　kě　yù,　shǐ　mín　xīn　bú　luàn.
NOT　SEE　CAN　DESIRE,　CAUSE　PEOPLE　HEART　NOT　DISORDER.

NOT SEEING DESIRABLE things ENSURES that the PEOPLE'S HEARTS will NOT be in DISORDER.

是　以　圣　人　之　治，
shì　yǐ　shèng-　rén　zhī　zhì,
BE　WHY　SAGACIOUS-　PERSON　[PART]　RULERSHIP,

This IS WHY the RULERSHIP OF the SAGE

虚　其　心，实　其　腹；
xū　qí　xīn,　shí　qí　fù;
EMPTY　THEIR　HEART,　FILL　THEIR　STOMACH;

EMPTIES the PEOPLE'S HEARTS, but FILLS THEIR STOMACHS;

弱　其　志，强　其　骨。

ruò　qí　zhì,　qiáng　qí　gǔ.
WEAKEN　THEIR　WILL,　STRENGTHEN　THEIR　BONE.

WEAKENS THEIR WILL, but STRENGTHENS THEIR BONES.

常　使　民　无　知　无　欲；

cháng　shǐ　mín　wú　zhī　wú　yù;
ALWAYS　CAUSE　PEOPLE　NOT　KNOW,　NOT　DESIRE;

The sage ALWAYS ENSURES that the PEOPLE do NOT KNOW and do NOT DESIRE;

使　夫　智　者　不　敢　为　也。

shǐ　fú　zhì　zhě　bù　gǎn　wéi　yě.
CAUSE　[PART]　INTELLECTUAL　[PART]　NOT　DARE　ACT　[PART].

He ENSURES that INTELLECTUALS will NOT DARE to INTERFERE.

为　无　为，

wéi　wú　wéi,
ACT　NOT　ACT,

He ENACTS NON-ACTION,

则　无　不　治。

zé　wú　bú　zhì.
YET　NOTHING　NOT　GOVERN.

YET there is NOTHING that is NOT GOVERNED.

道　冲，　而　用　之　或　不　盈。

dào　chōng,　ér　yòng　zhī　huò　bù　yíng.
DAO　EMPTY,　BUT　USE　IT　EVEN　NOT　FULL.

The DAO is EMPTY, BUT EVEN if one USES IT, it will NOT become FULL.

渊　兮；　似　万　物　之　宗。

yuān　xī;　sì　wàn　wù　zhī　zōng.
DEEP　[PART];　SEEM　TEN-THOUSAND　THING　[PART]　ANCESTOR.

It is DEEP; it SEEMS to be the ANCESTOR OF ALL THINGS.

挫　其　锐；　解　其　纷；

cuò　qí　ruì;　jiě　qí　fēn;
BLUNT　ITS　SHARP;　SEPARATE　ITS　ENTANGLED;

It BLUNTS the SHARP; it SEPARATES the ENTANGLED;

和　其　光；　同　其　尘。

hé　qí　guāng;　tóng　qí　chén.
DILUTE　ITS　BRIGHT;　UNITE　ITS　DUST.

It DILUTES the BRIGHT; it UNITES with DUST.

湛　兮，　似　或　存。

zhàn　xī,　sì　huò　cún.
PROFOUND　[PART],　SEEM　YET　PRESERVE.

It is PROFOUND, YET SEEMS always PRESERVED.

吾　不　知　谁　之　子；　象　帝　之　先。

wú　bù　zhī　shéi　zhī　zǐ;　xiàng　dì　zhī　xiān.
I　NOT　KNOW　WHO　[PART]　OFFSPRING;　SEEM　GOD　[PART]　PREDECESSOR.

I do NOT KNOW WHOSE OFFSPRING it is; it SEEMS to be the PREDECESSOR OF the GODS.

Chapter 5

天　地　不　仁;

tiān　dì　bù　rén;
HEAVEN　EARTH　NOT　KIND;

HEAVEN and EARTH are NOT KIND;

以　万　物　为　刍　狗。

yǐ　wàn　wù　wéi　chú　gǒu.
TAKE　TEN-THOUSAND　THING　TREAT　STRAW　DOG.

They TAKE ALL THINGS and TREAT them as STRAW DOGS.

圣　人　不　仁;

shèng-　rén　bù　rén;
SAGACIOUS-　PERSON　NOT　KIND;

The SAGE is NOT KIND;

以　百　姓　为　刍　狗。

yǐ　bǎi　xìng　wéi　chú　gǒu.
TAKE　HUNDRED　SURNAME　TREAT　STRAW　DOG.

He TAKES the PEOPLE and TREATS them as STRAW DOGS.

天　地　之　间,　其　犹　橐　籥　乎?

tiān　dì　zhī　jiān,　qí　yóu　tuó　yuè　hū?
HEAVEN　EARTH　[PART]　BETWEEN,　IT　LIKE　BELLOWS　[PART]?

Isn't the void BETWEEN HEAVEN and EARTH LIKE a BELLOWS?

虚　而　不　屈;　动　而　愈　出。

xū　ér　bù　qū;　dòng　ér　yù　chū.
EMPTY　BUT　NOT　DEFORM;　MOVE　BUT　MORE　EXTEND.

It is EMPTY BUT does NOT LOSE its FORM; one can MOVE it, BUT it EXTENDS all the MORE.

多　言　数　穷;　不　如　守　中。

duō　yán　shù　qióng;　bù　rú　shǒu　zhōng.
MANY　WORD　COUNT　POOR;　NOT　LIKE　MAINTAIN　CENTER.

MANY WORDS COUNT as FEW; it is BETTER to MAINTAIN the CENTER.

谷　神　不　死；是　谓　玄　牝。

gǔ　shén　bù　sǐ;　shì　wèi　xuán　pìn.

VALLEY　SPIRIT　NOT　DIE;　BE　CALL　MYSTERIOUS　FEMININE.

The SPIRIT of the VALLEY does NOT DIE; it IS CALLED "the MYSTERIOUS FEMININE."

玄　牝　之　门，是　谓　天　根。

xuán　pìn　zhī　mén,　shì　wèi　tiān　gēn.

MYSTERIOUS FEMININE　[PART]　GATE,　BE　CALL　HEAVEN　ROOT.

The GATE OF the MYSTERIOUS FEMININE IS CALLED "the ROOT of HEAVEN."

绵　绵　若　存；用　之　不　勤。

mián　mián　ruò　cún;　yòng　zhī　bù　qín.

CONTINUOUSLY　SEEM　PRESERVE;　USE　IT　NOT　EXHAUST.

It SEEMS to be CONTINUOUSLY PRESERVED; even if one USES IT, it will NOT be EXHAUSTED.

Chapter 7

天 长 地 久。

tiān   cháng,   dì   jiǔ.
HEAVEN   LONG,   EARTH   LONG-TIME.

HEAVEN is LONG-LASTING, the EARTH is LONG-LASTING.

天 地 所 以 能 长 久 者,

tiān   dì   suǒ   yǐ   néng   cháng   jiǔ   zhě,
HEAVEN   EARTH   REASON   CAN   LONG   LONG-TIME   [PART],

The REASON that HEAVEN and EARTH CAN be LONG-LASTING

以 其 不 自 生;

yǐ   qí   bú   zì   shēng;
BECAUSE   THEY   NOT   SELF   BORN;

Is THAT THEY were NOT BORN for the benefit of THEMSELVES;

故 能 长 生。

gù   néng   cháng   shēng.
THEREFORE   CAN   LONG   EXIST.

THEREFORE they CAN LONG EXIST.

是 以 圣 人 后 其 身, 而 身 先;

shì   yǐ   shèng-   rén   hòu   qí   shēn,   ér   shēn   xiān;
BE   WHY   SAGACIOUS-   PERSON   BEHIND   HIS   BODY,   BUT   BODY   FIRST;

This IS WHY the SAGE places HIMSELF BEHIND, YET HE is FIRST;

外 其 身, 而 身 存。

wài   qí   shēn,   ér   shēn   cún.
OUTSIDE   HIS   LIFE,   BUT   LIFE   PRESERVE.

He leaves HIS own LIFE OUT of consideration, BUT his LIFE is PRESERVED.

非　　以　　其　　无　　私　　邪？

fēi　　yǐ　　qí　　wú　　sī　　yé?

NOT　　BECAUSE　　HE　　NOT　　SELFISH　　[PART]?

Is this NOT BECAUSE HE is UNSELFISH?

故　　能　　成　　其　　私。

gù　　néng　　chéng　　qí　　sī.

THEREFORE　　CAN　　ACCOMPLISH　　HIS　　PURPOSE.

THEREFORE he CAN ACCOMPLISH HIS PURPOSE.

Chapter 8

上　善　若　水。

shàng　　shàn　　ruò　　shuǐ.
SUPREME　GOOD　LIKE　WATER.

The SUPREME GOOD is LIKE WATER.

水　善　利　万　物　而　不　争;

shuǐ　shàn　lì　wàn　wù　ér　bù　zhēng;
WATER　ADEPT　BENEFIT　TEN-THOUSAND　THING　BUT　NOT　CONTEND;

WATER is ADEPT at BENEFITTING ALL THINGS BUT does NOT CONTEND;

处　众　人　之　所　恶。

chǔ　zhòng　rén　zhī　suǒ　wù.
LOCATE　NUMEROUS　PERSON　[PART]　[PART]　LOATHE.

It is LOCATED in places LOATHED by the MULTITUDE.

故　几　于　道。

gù　jǐ　yú　dào.
THEREFORE　CLOSE　TO　DAO.

THEREFORE it is CLOSE TO the DAO.

居　善　地; 心　善　渊;

jū　shàn　dì;　xīn　shàn　yuān;
DWELL　EMPHASIZE　EARTH;　HEART　EMPHASIZE　DEEP-POOL;

In DWELLING, the sage EMPHASIZES the EARTH; in his HEART, he EMPHASIZES becoming like a DEEP POOL;

与　善　仁; 言　善　信;

yǔ　shàn　rén;　yán　shàn　xìn;
GIVE　EMPHASIZE BENEVOLENCE;　SPEAK　EMPHASIZE　TRUST;

In GIVING, he EMPHASIZES BENEVOLENCE; in SPEAKING, he EMPHASIZES TRUST;

政 善 治; 事 善 能;

zhèng   *shàn*   *zhì;*   *shì*   *shàn*   *néng;*
GOVERN   EMPHASIZE   RULE;   AFFAIR   EMPHASIZE   CAPABLE;

In GOVERNING, he EMPHASIZES effective RULERSHIP; in his AFFAIRS, he EMPHASIZES being CAPABLE;

动 善 时。

dòng   *shàn*   *shí.*
ACT   EMPHASIZE   TIME.

In ACTING, he EMPHASIZES TIMELINESS.

夫 唯 不 争, 故 无 尤。

fú   *wéi*   *bù*   *zhēng,*   *gù*   *wú*   *yóu.*
SINCE   NOT   CONTEND, THEREFORE   NOT   BLAME.

SINCE he does NOT CONTEND, he is NOT BLAMED.

Chapter 9

持　而　盈　之，　不　如　其　已；

chí　ér　yíng　zhī,　bù　rú　qí　yǐ;

PERSIST　AND　FILL　IT,　NOT　LIKE　IT　STOP;

To PERSIST in FILLING a VESSEL is NOT AS good as STOPPING;

揣　而　锐　之，　不　可　长　保。

chuǎi　ér　ruì　zhī,　bù　kě　cháng　bǎo.

STRIVE　AND　SHARPEN　IT,　NOT　CAN　LONG　RETAIN.

If one keeps STRIVING to SHARPEN a KNIFE, it CANNOT LONG REMAIN sharp.

金　玉　满　堂，　莫　之　能　守。

jīn　yù　mǎn　táng,　mò　zhī　néng　shǒu.

GOLD　JADE　FULL　CHAMBER,　NOT　IT　POSSIBLE　DEFEND.

If one's CHAMBER is FULL of GOLD and JADE, it will be IMPOSSIBLE to DEFEND IT.

富　贵　而　骄，　自　遗　其　咎。

fù　guì　ér　jiāo,　zì　yí　qí　jiù.

WEALTH　RANK　AND　ARROGANT,　SELF　HAND-DOWN　ONE'S　PUNISHMENT.

To acquire WEALTH and RANK AND be ARROGANT is to HAND DOWN ONE'S own PUNISHMENT.

成　功　身　退：　天　之　道　也。

chéng　gōng　shēn　tuì:　tiān　zhī　dào　yě.

ACCOMPLISH　MERITORIOS-ACT　BODY　WITHDRAW:　HEAVEN　[PART]　DAO　[PART].

To ACCOMPLISH MERITORIOUS ACTS and then WITHDRAW: this is the DAO OF HEAVEN.

载	营	魄	抱	一，	能	无	离	乎？
zài	yíng	pò	bào	yī,	néng	wú	lí	hū?
CARRY	BODY	SOUL	HOLD	ONE,	CAN	NOT	SEPARATE	[PART]?

In CARRYING BODY and SOUL and HOLDING them as ONE, CAN you REFRAIN from SEPARATING them?

专	气	致	柔，	能	如	婴	儿	乎？
zhuān	qì	zhì	róu,	néng	rú	yīng-	ér	hū?
CONCENTRATE	SPIRIT	ACHIEVE	PLIANT,	CAN	LIKE	BABY-	CHILD	[PART]?

In CONCENTRATING your SPIRIT and ACHIEVING PLIANCY, CAN you become LIKE a BABY?

涤	除	玄	鉴，	能	无	疵	乎？
dí-	chú,	xuán	jiàn,	néng	wú	cī	hū?
CLEANSE-	ELIMINATE	PROFOUND	CONTEMPLATE,	CAN	NOT	FLAW	[PART]?

In CLEANSING your mind and CONTEMPLATING the PROFOUND, CAN you remain WITHOUT FLAW?

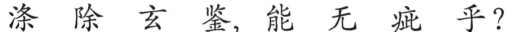

爱	民	治	国，	能	无	为	乎？
ài	mín	zhì	guó,	néng	wú	wéi	hū?
LOVE	PEOPLE	RULE	COUNTRY,	CAN	NOT	ACT	[PART]?

In LOVING the PEOPLE and RULING the COUNTRY, CAN you REFRAIN from ACTING?

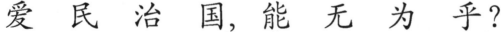

天	门	开	阖，	能	为	雌	乎？
tiān	mén	kāi	hé,	néng	wéi	cí	hū?
HEAVEN	GATE	OPEN	SHUT,	CAN	SERVE-AS	FEMININE	[PART]?

When the GATES of HEAVEN OPEN and SHUT, CAN you SERVE in a FEMININE role?

明	白	四	达，	能	无	知	乎？
míng	bái,	sì	dá,	néng	wú	zhī	hū?
UNDERSTAND,		FOUR	COMPREHEND,	CAN	NOT	KNOW	[PART]?

In UNDERSTANDING the FOUR things, CAN you remain WITHOUT KNOWING?

生 之 畜 之, 生 而 不 有,

shēng *zhī* *xù* *zhī,* *shēng* *ér* *bù* *yǒu,*

PRODUCE IT GROW IT, PRODUCE BUT NOT POSSESS,

PRODUCE and allow to GROW, PRODUCE BUT do NOT POSSESS,

为 而 不 恃, 长 而 不 宰:

wéi *ér* *bú* *shì,* *cháng* *ér* *bù* *zǎi:*

ACT BUT NOT DEPEND, PROMOTE BUT NOT CONTROL:

ACT BUT do NOT DEPEND, PROMOTE BUT do NOT CONTROL:

是 谓 玄 德。

shì *wèi* *xuán* *dé.*

BE CALL PROFOUND VIRTUE.

This IS CALLED "PROFOUND VIRTUE."

Chapter 11

三 十 辐 共 一 毂;

sān- shí fú gòng yì gǔ;

THREE- TEN SPOKE SHARE ONE HUB;

THIRTY SPOKES SHARE ONE HUB;

当 其 无, 有 车 之 用。

dāng qí wú, yōu chē zhī yòng.

GIVEN THEIR NOTHINGNESS, HAVE CART [PART] USE.

GIVEN the EMPTY spaces, one HAS the USE OF the CART.

埏 埴 以 为 器;

shān zhí yǐ wéi qì;

CLAY FILL TO SERVE-AS VESSEL;

CLAY is SHAPED TO SERVE AS a VESSEL;

当 其 无, 有 器 之 用。

dāng qí wú, yǒu qì zhī yòng.

GIVEN ITS NOTHINGNESS, HAVE VESSEL [PART] USE.

GIVEN the EMPTY space, one HAS the USE OF the VESSEL.

凿 户 牖 以 为 室;

záo hù yǒu yǐ wéi shì;

CUT DOOR WINDOW TO SERVE-AS CHAMBER;

CUT out DOORS and WINDOWS TO CREATE a CHAMBER;

当 其 无, 有 室 之 用。

dāng qí wú, yǒu shì zhī yòng.

GIVEN THEIR NOTHINGNESS, HAVE CHAMBER [PART] USE.

GIVEN the EMPTY spaces, one HAS the USE OF the CHAMBER.

故　有　之　以　为　利;
gù　yǒu　zhī　yǐ　wéi　lì;
THEREFORE　HAVE　IT　[PART]　SERVE-AS　BENEFIT;

THEREFORE HAVING PROVIDES BENEFIT;

无　之　以　为　用。
wú　zhī　yǐ　wéi　yòng.
NOT　IT　[PART]　SERVE-AS　USE.

NOTHINGNESS PROVIDES USE.

五　色　令　人　目　盲。

wǔ　sè　lìng　rén　mù　máng.
FIVE　COLOR　CAUSE　PERSON　EYE　BLIND.

The FIVE COLORS CAUSE the EYE to be BLINDED.

五　音　令　人　耳　聋。

wǔ　yīn　lìng　rén　ěr　lóng.
FIVE　SOUND　CAUSE　PERSON　EAR　DEAF.

The FIVE SOUNDS CAUSE the EAR to become DEAF.

五　味　令　人　口　爽。

wǔ　wèi　lìng　rén　kǒu　shuǎng.
FIVE　FLAVOR　CAUSE　PERSON　MOUTH　RAW.

The FIVE FLAVORS CAUSE the MOUTH to become RAW.

驰　骋　畋　猎，令　人　心　发　狂。

chí　chěng　tián　liè,　lìng　rén　xīn　fā　kuáng.
GALLOP　HUNT,　CAUSE　PERSON　HEART　EMIT　MAD.

GALLOPING and HUNTING CAUSE the HEART to GO MAD.

难　得　之　货，令　人　行　妨。

nán　dé　zhī　huò,　lìng　rén　xíng　fáng.
DIFFICULT　OBTAIN　[PART]　COMMODITY,　CAUSE　PERSON　CONDUCT　HINDER.

RARE COMMODITIES CAUSE a PERSON'S CONDUCT to be HINDERED.

是　以　圣　人　为　腹；不　为　目。

shì　yǐ　shèng-　rén　wéi　fù;　bù　wéi　mù.
BE　WHY　SAGACIOUS-　PERSON　ACT　STOMACH;　NOT　ACT　EYE.

This IS WHY the SAGE ACTS emphasizing the STOMACH, NOT the EYE.

故　去　彼　取　此。

gù　qù　bǐ　qǔ　cǐ.
THEREFORE　GO　THAT　TAKE　THIS.

THEREFORE he LEAVES THAT and TAKES THIS.

Chapter 13

宠　辱　若　惊；贵　大　患　若　身。

chǒng　rǔ　ruò　jīng;　guì　dà　huàn　ruò　shēn.

FAVOR　DISGRACE　SEEM　FRIGHTEN;　APPRAISE　GREAT　CALAMITY　AS　LIFE.

FAVOR and DISGRACE SEEM FRIGHTENING; APPRAISE GREAT CALAMITY AS part of LIFE.

何　谓　宠　辱　若　惊？

hé　wèi　chǒng　rǔ　ruò　jīng?

WHY　SAY　FAVOR　DISGRACE　SEEM　FRIGHTEN?

WHY is it SAID that FAVOR and DISGRACE SEEM FRIGHTENING?

宠　为　下：

chǒng　wéi　xià:

FAVOR　ACT　INFERIOR:

FAVOR ACTS in an INFERIOR manner:

得　之　若　惊；失　之　若　惊。

dé　zhī　ruò　jīng;　shī　zhī　ruò　jīng.

OBTAIN　IT　SEEM　FRIGHTEN;　LOSE　IT　SEEM　FRIGHTEN.

To OBTAIN IT SEEMS FRIGHTENING; to LOSE IT SEEMS FRIGHTENING.

是　谓　宠　辱　若　惊。

shì　wèi　chǒng　rǔ　ruò　jīng.

BE　SAY　FAVOR　DISGRACE　SEEM　FRIGHTEN.

Therefore it IS SAID that FAVOR and DISGRACE SEEM FRIGHTENING.

何　谓　贵　大　患　若　身？

hé　wèi　guì　dà　huàn　ruò　shēn?

WHY　SAY　APPRAISE　GREAT　CALAMITY　AS　LIFE?

WHY is it SAID that one should APPRAISE GREAT CALAMITY AS part of LIFE?

吾　所　以　有　大　患　者，为　吾

wú　suǒ　yǐ　yǒu　dà　huàn　zhě,　wéi　wú

I　REASON　　HAVE　GREAT　CALAMITY　[PART],　BECAUSE　I

有　身；

yǒu　shēn;

HAVE　LIFE;

The REASON I EXPERIENCE GREAT CALAMITY is THAT I HAVE LIFE;

及　吾　无　身，吾　有　何　患？

jí　wú　wú　shēn,　wú　yǒu　hé　huàn?

IF　I　NOT　LIFE,　I　HAVE　WHAT　CALAMITY?

IF I did NOT have LIFE, WHAT CALAMITY could I EXPERIENCE?

故　贵　以　身　为　天　下，

gù　guì　yǐ　shēn　wéi　tiān　xià,

THEREFORE　VALUE　[PART]　LIFE　ACT　HEAVEN　UNDER,

THEREFORE those who VALUE LIFE while ACTING UNDER HEAVEN

若　可　寄　天　下。

ruò　kě　jì　tiān　xià.

THEN　CAN　ENTRUST　HEAVEN　UNDER.

CAN be ENTRUSTED with all things UNDER HEAVEN.

爱　以　身　为　天　下，

ài　yǐ　shēn　wéi　tiān　xià,

LOVE　[PART]　LIFE　ACT　HEAVEN　UNDER,

Those who LOVE LIFE while ACTING UNDER HEAVEN

若　可　托　天　下。

ruò　kě　tuō　tiān　xià.

THEN　CAN　ENTRUST　HEAVEN　UNDER.

CAN be ENTRUSTED with all things UNDER HEAVEN.

视　　之　　不　　见，　名　　曰　　夷。
shì　　*zhī*　　*bú*　　*jiàn,*　　*míng*　　*yuē*　　*yí.*
WATCH　　IT　　NOT　　SEE,　　NAME　　CALL　　ERASE.

WATCHED for but NOT SEEN, its NAME IS "ERASED."

听　　之　　不　　闻，　名　　曰　　希。
tīng　　*zhī*　　*bù*　　*wén,*　　*míng*　　*yuē*　　*xī.*
LISTEN　　IT　　NOT　　HEAR,　　NAME　　CALL　　RARE.

LISTENED for but NOT HEARD, its NAME IS "RARE."

搏　　之　　不　　得，　名　　曰　　微。
bó　　*zhī*　　*bù*　　*dé,*　　*míng*　　*yuē*　　*wēi.*
GRASP　　IT　　NOT　　REACH,　　NAME　　CALL　　ABSTRUSE.

GRASPED at but NOT REACHED, its NAME IS "ABSTRUSE."

此　　三　　者　　不　　可　　致　　诘；　故　　混
cǐ　　*sān*　　*zhě*　　*bù*　　*kě*　　*zhì*　　*jié;*　　*gù*　　*hùn*
THESE　　THREE　　[PART]　　NOT　　CAN　　FATHOM;　　THEREFORE　　MIX

为　　一。
wéi　　*yī.*
AS　　ONE.

THESE THREE are UNFATHOMABLE; THEREFORE they MIX together AS ONE.

其　　上　　不　　皦；　其　　下　　不　　昧。
qí　　*shàng*　　*bù*　　*jiǎo;*　　*qí*　　*xià*　　*bú*　　*mèi.*
IT　　ABOVE　　NOT　　BRIGHT;　　IT　　BELOW　　NOT　　DARK.

ABOVE the ONE there is NO BRIGHTNESS; BELOW IT there is NO DARKNESS.

绳	绳	兮;	不	可	名;	复	归	于
shéng	*shéng*	*xī;*	*bù*	*kě*	*míng;*	*fù-*	*guī*	*yú*
RESTRICT		[PART];	NOT	CAN	NAME;	TURN-	RETURN	TO

无	物。
wú	*wù.*
NOT	MATERIAL.

It is RESTRICTED; it CANNOT be NAMED; it RETURNS TO the IMMATERIAL.

是	谓	无	状	之	状;
shì	*wèi*	*wú*	*zhuàng*	*zhī*	*zhuàng;*
BE	CALL	NOT	FORM	[PART]	FORM;

It IS CALLED "the FORMLESS FORM;

无	物	之	象;
wú	*wù*	*zhī*	*xiàng;*
NOT	MATERIAL	[PART]	IMAGE;

the IMAGE of the IMMATERIAL."

是	谓	恍	惚。
shì	*wèi*	*huǎng*	*hū.*
BE	CALL		DIM.

It IS CALLED "DIM."

迎	之	不	见	其	首;	随	之	不	见
yíng	*zhī*	*bú*	*jiàn*	*qí*	*shǒu;*	*suí*	*zhī*	*bú*	*jiàn*
FACE	IT	NOT	SEE	ITS	BEGINNING;	FOLLOW	IT	NOT	SEE

其	后。
qí	*hòu.*
ITS	END.

If one FACES IT, ITS BEGINNING CANNOT be SEEN; if one FOLLOWS IT, ITS END CANNOT be SEEN.

执　　古　　之　　道，　以　　御　　今　　之　　有。

zhí　　gǔ　　zhī　　dào,　　yǐ　　yù　　jīn　　zhī　　yǒu.
HOLD　ANCIENT　[PART]　DAO,　TO　HANDLE　TODAY　[PART]　AFFAIR.

HOLD fast to the ANCIENT DAO TO HANDLE TODAY'S AFFAIRS.

能　　知　　古　　始，　是　　谓　　道　　纪。

néng　　zhī　　gǔ　　shǐ,　　shì　　wèi　　dào　　jì.
CAN　KNOW　ANCIENT　BEGINNING,　BE　CALL　DAO　LAW.

KNOWING the ANCIENT BEGINNING IS CALLED "the LAW of the DAO."

古　之　善　为　道　者，微　妙　玄　通，

gǔ　　zhī　　shàn　　wéi　　dào　　zhě,　　wēi　　miào　　xuán　　tōng,

ANCIENT　[PART]　ADEPT　ACT　DAO　[PART],　SUBTLE　　PROFOUND,

The ANCIENT ONES ADEPT at ENACTING the DAO were SUBTLE and PROFOUND,

深　不　可　识。

shēn　　bù　　kě　　shí.

DEEP　NOT　CAN　KNOW.

So DEEP that they CANNOT be KNOWN.

夫　唯　不　可　识，故　强　为　其　容：

fú　　wéi　　bù　　kě　　shí,　　gù　　qiáng　　wèi　　zhī　　róng:

SINCE　NOT　CAN　KNOW,　THEREFORE　MUST　FOR　THEM　DESCRIBE:

SINCE they CANNOT be KNOWN, one MUST DESCRIBE THEM:

豫　兮，若　冬　涉　川；

yù　　xī,　　ruò　　dōng　　shè　　chuān;

CAUTIOUS　[PART],　LIKE　WINTER　FORD　RIVER;

CAUTIOUS, they were LIKE someone FORDING a RIVER in WINTER;

犹　兮，若　畏　四　邻；

yóu　　xī,　　ruò　　wèi　　sì　　lín;

VIGILANT　[PART],　LIKE　FEAR　FOUR　NEIGHBOR;

VIGILANT, they were LIKE someone who FEARS ENEMIES on ALL sides;

俨　兮　其　若　容；

yǎn　　xī　・　qí　　ruò　　róng;

DIGNIFIED　[PART]　THEY　LIKE　GUEST;

DIGNIFIED, THEY were LIKE GUESTS;

涣　兮　其　若　凌　释；

huàn　*xī*　*qí*　*ruò*　*líng*　*shì;*

EVANESCENT　[PART]　THEY　LIKE　ICE　MELT;

EVANESCENT, THEY were LIKE MELTING ICE;

敦　兮　其　若　朴；

dūn　*xī*　*qí*　*ruò*　*pǔ;*

SINCERE　[PART]　THEY　LIKE　BLOCK-OF-WOOD;

SINCERE, THEY were LIKE a BLOCK OF WOOD;

旷　兮　其　若　谷；

kuàng　*xī*　*qí*　*ruò*　*gǔ;*

VAST　[PART]　THEY　LIKE　VALLEY;

VAST, THEY were LIKE a VALLEY;

混　兮　其　若　浊。

hùn　*xī*　*qí*　*ruò*　*zhuó.*

TURBULENT　[PART]　THEY　LIKE　SWIRLING-WATER.

TURBULENT, THEY were LIKE SWIRLING WATER.

孰　能　浊　以　静　之　徐　清？

shú　*néng*　*zhuó*　*yǐ*　*jìng*　*zhī*　*xú*　*qīng?*

WHO　ENABLE　TURBULENT　TAKE　CALM　[PART]　SLOW　TRANQUILITY?

WHO ENABLES the TURBULENT to TAKE on the SLOW TRANQUILITY OF CALM?

孰　能　安　以　动　之　徐　生？

shú　*néng*　*ān*　*yǐ*　*dòng*　*zhī*　*xú*　*shēng?*

WHO　ENABLE　CALM　TAKE　MOTION　[PART]　SLOW　BIRTH?

WHO ENABLES the CALM to TAKE on the SLOW BIRTH OF MOTION?

保　此　道　者，　不　欲　盈。
bǎo　*cǐ*　*dào*　*zhě,*　*bú*　*yù*　*yíng.*
UPHOLD　THIS　DAO　[PART],　NOT　DESIRE　OVERFULL.

Those WHO UPHOLD THIS DAO do NOT DESIRE OVERFULLNESS.

夫　唯　不　盈，　故　能　蔽　而　新　成。
fú　*wéi*　*bù*　*yíng,*　*gù*　*néng*　*bì*　*ér*　*xīn*　*chéng.*
SINCE　　NOT　OVERFULL,　THEREFORE　CAN　OLD　BUT　NEW　ACHIEVE.

SINCE they are NOT OVERFULL, they CAN use the OLD BUT ACHIEVE the NEW.

Chapter 16

致　虚　极;　守　静　笃。

zhì　xū　jí;　shǒu　jìng　dǔ.

STRIVE　EMPTY　UTMOST;　MAINTAIN　TRANQUIL　SINCERE.

STRIVE to the UTMOST to be EMPTY; MAINTAIN TRANQUILITY and SINCERITY.

万　物　并　作;　吾　以　观　复。

wàn　wù　bìng　zuò;　wú　yǐ　guān　fù.

TEN-THOUSAND THING　SIDE-BY-SIDE DEVELOP;　I　[PART]　WATCH　RETURN.

ALL THINGS DEVELOP SIDE BY SIDE; I WATCH them RETURN.

夫　物　芸　芸，　各　复　归　其　根。

fú　wù　yún　yún,　gè　fù-　guī　qí　gēn.

THOUGH　THING　PROFUSION,　EACH　TURN-　RETURN　ITS　ROOT.

THOUGH THINGS exist in PROFUSION, EACH RETURNS to ITS ROOT.

归　根　曰　静;　静　曰　复　命。

guī　gēn　yuē　jìng;　jìng　yuē　fù　mìng.

RETURN　ROOT　CALL　TRANQUIL;　TRANQUIL　CALL　RETURN　LIFE.

RETURNING to the ROOT is CALLED "TRANQUILITY;" TRANQUILITY is CALLED "RETURNING to LIFE."

复　命　曰　常;　知　常　曰　明。

fù　mìng　yuē　cháng;　zhī　cháng　yuē　míng.

RETURN　LIFE　CALL　UNCHANGING;　KNOW　UNCHANGING　CALL　BRIGHT.

RETURNING to LIFE is CALLED "the UNCHANGING;" to KNOW the UNCHANGING is called "BRIGHTNESS."

不　知　常，　妄　作　凶。

bù　zhī　cháng,　wàng　zuò　xiōng.

NOT　KNOW　UNCHANGING,　RASHLY　PRODUCE　DISASTER.

NOT to KNOW the UNCHANGING is to RASHLY BRING about DISASTER.

知　常　容；容　乃　公；

zhī　cháng　róng;　róng　nǎi　gōng;
KNOW　UNCHANGING　TOLERANT;　TOLERANT　SO　JUST;

To KNOW the UNCHANGING is to be TOLERANT; if one is TOLERANT one will be JUST;

公　乃　全；全　乃　天；

gōng　nǎi　quán;　quán　nǎi　tiān;
JUST　SO　WHOLE;　WHOLE　SO　HEAVEN;

If one is JUST one will be WHOLE; if one is WHOLE one will understand HEAVEN;

天　乃　道；道　乃　久；

tiān　nǎi　dào;　dào　nǎi　jiǔ;
HEAVEN　SO　DAO;　DAO　SO　LONG;

If one understands HEAVEN one will have the DAO; if one has the DAO one will LONG continue;

没　身　不　殆。

mò　shēn　bú　dài.
END　LIFE　NOT　HARM.

Unto the END of LIFE there will be NO HARM.

Chapter 17

太　　上，　不　　知　　有　　之；
tài　　shàng,　bù　　zhī　　yǒu　　zhī;
BEST　　RULER,　NOT　　KNOW　　EXIST　　HIM;

As for the BEST RULER, the people do NOT KNOW that HE EXISTS;

其　　次，　亲　　而　　誉　　之；
qí　　cì,　　qīn　　ér　　yù　　zhī;
ITS　　NEXT,　CLOSE　　AND　　PRAISE　　HIM;

As for the NEXT best, they are CLOSE to him AND PRAISE HIM;

其　　次，　畏　　之；
qí　　cì,　　wèi　　zhī;
ITS　　NEXT,　FEAR　　HIM;

As for the NEXT best, they FEAR HIM;

其　　次，　侮　　之。
qí　　cì,　　wǔ　　zhī.
ITS　　NEXT,　SCORN　　HIM.

As for the NEXT best, they SCORN HIM.

信　　不　　足　　焉，　有　　不　　信　　焉。
xìn　　bù　　zú　　yān,　yǒu　　bú　　xìn　　yān.
TRUSTWORTHINESS NOT　　SUFFICIENT　[PART],　EXIST　　NOT　　TRUST　　[PART].

If the ruler is NOT SUFFICIENTLY TRUSTWORTHY, there will BE DISTRUST.

悠　　兮；　其　　贵　　言。
yōu　　xī;　　qí　　guì　　yán.
LEISURELY　[PART];　HE　　TREASURE　SPEECH.

The best ruler acts in a LEISURELY manner; HE regards SPEECH as a TREASURE not to be disbursed.

功　成，事　遂，

gōng　chéng,　shì　suì,

MERITORIOUS-ACT ACHIEVE,　AFFAIR　ACCOMPLISH,

When his MERITORIOUS ACTS are ACHIEVED and his AFFAIRS are ACCOMPLISHED

百　姓　皆　谓 "我　自　然"。

bǎi　xìng　jiē　wèi　wǒ　zì　rán.

HUNDRED SURNAME　ALL　SAY　I　SELF　THUS.

The PEOPLE ALL SAY: "I have achieved this MYSELF."

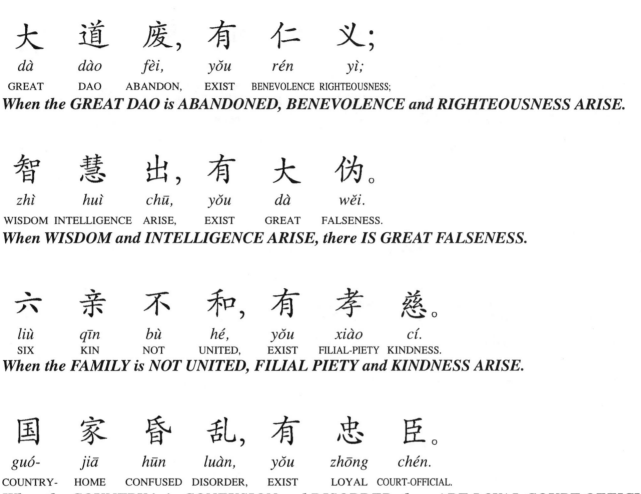

Chapter 18

大　道　废，有　仁　义;
dà　dào　fèi,　yǒu　rén　yì;
GREAT　DAO　ABANDON,　EXIST　BENEVOLENCE RIGHTEOUSNESS;
When the GREAT DAO is ABANDONED, BENEVOLENCE and RIGHTEOUSNESS ARISE.

智　慧　出，有　大　伪。
zhì　huì　chū,　yǒu　dà　wěi.
WISDOM INTELLIGENCE　ARISE,　EXIST　GREAT　FALSENESS.
When WISDOM and INTELLIGENCE ARISE, there IS GREAT FALSENESS.

六　亲　不　和，有　孝　慈。
liù　qīn　bù　hé,　yǒu　xiào　cí.
SIX　KIN　NOT　UNITED,　EXIST　FILIAL-PIETY KINDNESS.
When the FAMILY is NOT UNITED, FILIAL PIETY and KINDNESS ARISE.

国　家　昏　乱，有　忠　臣。
guó-　jiā　hūn　luàn,　yǒu　zhōng　chén.
COUNTRY-　HOME　CONFUSED DISORDER,　EXIST　LOYAL　COURT-OFFICIAL.
When the COUNTRY is in CONFUSION and DISORDER, there ARE LOYAL COURT OFFICIALS.

Chapter 19

绝　圣，弃　智：民　利　百　倍；

jué　shèng,　qì　zhì:　mín　lì　bǎi　bèi.

ABANDON SAGACIOUS,　REJECT　WISDOM:　PEOPLE　BENEFIT　HUNDRED　TIME.

ABANDON the SAGACIOUS, REJECT WISDOM: the BENEFIT for the PEOPLE will be a HUNDRED TIMES greater.

绝　仁，弃　义：

jué　rén,　qì　yì:

ABANDON BENEVOLENCE,　REJECT　RIGHTEOUSNESS:

ABANDON BENEVOLENCE and REJECT RIGHTEOUSNESS:

民　复　孝　慈。

mín　fù　xiào　cí.

PEOPLE　RETURN　FILIAL-PIETY　KINDNESS.

The PEOPLE will RETURN to FILIAL PIETY and KINDNESS.

绝　巧，弃　利：盗　贼　无　有。

jué　qiǎo,　qì　lì:　dào　zéi　wú　yǒu.

ABANDON CLEVERNESS,　REJECT　ADVANTAGE: BANDIT　THIEF　NOT　EXIST.

ABANDON CLEVERNESS and REJECT ADVANTAGE: there will BE NO BANDITS and THIEVES.

此　三　者　以　为　文　不　足。

cǐ　sān　zhě　yǐ　wéi　wén　bù　zú.

THESE　THREE　[PART]　TAKE　AS　PRINCIPLE　NOT　SUFFICIENT.

To TAKE THESE THREE AS a guiding PRINCIPLE is NOT SUFFICIENT.

故　令　有　所　属。

gù　lìng　yǒu　suǒ　shǔ.

THEREFORE　MUST　EXIST　[PART]　SUBORDINATE.

THEREFORE there MUST BE SUBORDINATION.

见　　素　　抱　　朴;
jiàn　　sù　　bào　　pǔ;
SEE　　PLAIN　　EMBRACE　　SIMPLE;

SEE the PLAIN and EMBRACE the SIMPLE;

少　　私　　寡　　欲。
shǎo　　sī　　guǎ　　yù.
REDUCE　　SELFISH　　FEW　　DESIRE.

REDUCE SELFISHNESS and have FEW DESIRES.

绝　　学　　无　　忧。
jué　　xué　　wú　　yōu.
ABANDON　　SCHOLARSHIP　　NOT　　WORRY.

ABANDON SCHOLARSHIP and there will be NO WORRY.

唯　之　与　阿：相　去　几　何？

wěi　*zhī*　*yǔ*　*ā:*　*xiāng*　*qù*　*jǐ*　*hé?*

"YES"　IT　AND　"NO:"　MUTUALLY　GO　HOW-MUCH　HOW?

AGREEMENT AND DISAGREEMENT: HOW MUCH do they MUTUALLY DIFFER?

善　之　与　恶：相　去　若　何？

shàn　*zhī*　*yǔ*　*è:*　*xiāng*　*qù*　*ruò*　*hé?*

GOOD　IT　AND　EVIL:　MUTUALLY　GO　AS　HOW?

GOOD AND EVIL: HOW do they MUTUALLY DIFFER?

人　之　所　畏，不　可　不　畏。

rén　*zhī*　*suǒ*　*wèi,*　*bù*　*kě*　*bú*　*wèi.*

PEOPLE　[PART]　WHAT　FEAR,　NOT　CAN　NOT　FEAR.

As for WHAT PEOPLE FEAR, it is IMPOSSIBLE NOT to FEAR it.

荒　兮；其　未　央　哉。

huāng　*xī;*　*qí*　*wèi*　*yāng*　*zāi.*

DESOLATE　[PART];　IT　NOT　END　[PART].

There is DESOLATION; IT is UNENDING.

众　人　熙　熙，

zhòng　*rén*　*xī*　*xī,*

NUMEROUS　PERSON　HAPPY,

The MULTITUDE are HAPPY,

如　享　太　牢；如　春　登　台。

rú　*xiǎng*　*tài*　*láo;*　*rú*　*chūn*　*dēng*　*tái.*

AS　ENJOY　SUPREME　OX-SACRIFICE;　AS　SPRING　CLIMB　TERRACE.

AS if ENJOYING the SUPREME feast of the SACRIFICIAL OX; AS if CLIMBING TERRACES in the SPRING.

我　独　泊　兮，　其　未　兆。
wǒ　dú　bó　xī,　qí　wèi　zhào.
I　ALONE　WAVER　[PART],　IT　NOT　TRACE.

I ALONE WAVER WITHOUT leaving a TRACE.

沌　沌　兮，　如　婴　儿　之　未　孩。
dùn　dùn　xī,　rú　yīng-　ér　zhī　wèi　hái.
UNKNOWING　[PART],　LIKE　BABY-　CHILD　[PART]　NOT　LAUGH.

I am UNKNOWING, LIKE a BABY that has NEVER yet LAUGHED.

累　累　兮，　若　无　所　归。
lèi　lèi　xī,　ruò　wú　suǒ　guī.
TIRED　[PART],　AS　NOT　WHERE　RETURN.

I am TIRED, AS if there were NOWHERE to RETURN to.

众　人　皆　有　馀，　而　我　独　若　遗。
zhòng　rén　jiē　yǒu　yú,　ér　wǒ　dú　ruò　yí.
NUMEROUS　PERSON　ALL　HAVE　EXCESS,　BUT　I　ALONE　SEEM　LOSE.

The MULTITUDE ALL HAVE everything in EXCESS, BUT I ALONE SEEM to have LOST everything.

我　愚　人　之　心　也　哉！
wǒ　yú　rén　zhī　xīn　yě　zāi!
I　FOOLISH　PERSON　[PART]　HEART　[PART]　[PART]!

O MY FOOLISH HEART!

俗　人　昭　昭；　我　独　昏　昏。
sú　rén　zhāo　zhāo;　wǒ　dú　hūn　hūn.
COMMON　PEOPLE　CLEAR;　I　ALONE　MUDDLED.

The COMMON PEOPLE are CLEAR; I ALONE am MUDDLED.

俗　人　察　察;　我　独　闷　闷。
sú　rén　chá　chá;　wǒ　dú　mèn　mèn.
COMMON　PEOPLE　CLEVER;　I　ALONE　DULL.

The COMMON PEOPLE are CLEVER; I ALONE am DULL.

澹　兮,　其　若　海;　飂　兮,　若　无　止。
dàn　xī,　qí　ruò　hǎi;　liáo　xī,　ruò　wú　zhǐ.
DISTANT　[PART],　IT　LIKE　SEA;　STORM　[PART],　LIKE　NOT　STOP.

I feel DISTANT, LIKE the SEA; STORMY, LIKE a gale that NEVER STOPS.

众　人　皆　有　以,　而　我　独　顽　且
zhòng　rén　jiē　yǒu　yǐ,　ér　wǒ　dú　wán　qiě
MULTITUDE　PERSON　ALL　HAVE　TAKE,　BUT　I　ALONE　STUPID　AND

鄙。
bǐ.
LOWLY.

The MULTITUDE ALL HAVE tasks to TAKE up, BUT I ALONE am STUPID AND LOWLY.

我　独　异　于　人,　而　贵　食　母。
wǒ　dú　yì　yú　rén,　ér　guì　shí　mǔ.
I　ALONE　DIFFERENT　FROM　PERSON,　BUT　VALUE　SUSTENANCE　MOTHER.

I ALONE am DIFFERENT FROM OTHERS, BUT I VALUE the MOTHER of SUSTENANCE.

Chapter 21

孔　德　之　容，惟　道　是　从。

kǒng　dé　zhī　róng,　wéi　dào　shì　cóng.

GREAT　VIRTUE　[PART]　CONTENT,　ONLY　DAO　BE　FOLLOW.

The CONTENT OF GREAT VIRTUE IS to FOLLOW ONLY the DAO.

道　之　为　物，惟　恍　惟　惚。

dào　zhī　wéi　wù,　wéi　huǎng　wéi　hū.

DAO　[PART]　ACT　SUBSTANCE,　ONLY　DIM　ONLY　FAINT.

Insofar as the DAO ACTS as SUBSTANCE, it is ONLY DIM, ONLY FAINT.

惚　兮　恍　兮，其　中　有　象；

hū　xī　huǎng　xī,　qí　zhōng　yǒu　xiàng;

DIM　[PART]　FAINT　[PART],　ITS　INTERIOR　EXIST　IMAGE;

DIM and FAINT, but WITHIN IT there IS an IMAGE;

恍　兮　惚　兮，其　中　有　物；

huǎng　xī　hū　xī,　qí　zhōng　yǒu　wù;

FAINT　[PART]　DIM　[PART],　ITS　INTERIOR　EXIST　SUBSTANCE;

FAINT and DIM, but WITHIN IT there IS SUBSTANCE;

窈　兮　冥　兮，其　中　有　精；

yǎo　xī　míng　xī,　qí　zhōng　yǒu　jīng;

SECLUDED　[PART]　DARK　[PART],　ITS　INTERIOR　EXIST　ESSENCE;

SECLUDED and DARK, but WITHIN IT there IS ESSENCE;

其　精　甚　真；其　中　有　信。

qí　jīng　shèn　zhēn;　qí　zhōng　yǒu　xìn.

ITS　ESSENCE　VERY　REAL;　ITS　INTERIOR　EXIST　BELIEF.

ITS ESSENCE is VERY REAL; WITHIN IT there IS BELIEF.

自　今　及　古，其　名　不　去；
zì　jīn　jí　gǔ,　qí　míng　bú　qù;
FROM　NOW　UNTIL　ANCIENT,　ITS　NAME　NOT　GO;

FROM ANCIENT times UNTIL NOW, ITS NAME has NOT DISAPPEARED;

以　阅　众　甫。
yǐ　yuè　zhòng　fǔ.
USE　OBSERVE　NUMEROUS　FATHER.

USE it to OBSERVE the FATHER of the NUMEROUS things.

吾　何　以　知　众　甫　之　状　哉？
wú　hé　yǐ　zhī　zhòng　fǔ　zhī　zhuàng　zāi?
I　HOW　[PART]　KNOW　NUMEROUS　FATHER　[PART]　CONDITION　[PART]?

HOW do I KNOW the CONDITION OF the FATHER of the NUMEROUS things?

以　此。
yǐ　cǐ.
USE　THIS.

I USE THIS dao.

Chapter 22

曲　则　全；　枉　则　直；

qū　zé　quán;　wǎng　zé　zhí;

CROOKED　YET　WHOLE;　TWISTED　YET　STRAIGHT;

CROOKED YET WHOLE; TWISTED YET STRAIGHT;

洼　则　盈；　敝　则　新；

wā　zé　yíng;　bì　zé　xīn;

FLAT　YET　FULL;　OLD　YET　NEW;

FLAT YET FULL; OLD YET NEW;

少　则　得；　多　则　惑。

shǎo　zé　dé;　duō　zé　huò.

LITTLE　YET　GAIN;　MUCH　YET　CONFUSED.

One can possess LITTLE, YET GAIN; one can possess MUCH, YET feel CONFUSED.

是　以　圣　人　抱　一，　为　天　下　式。

shì　yǐ　shèng-　rén　bào　yī,　wèi　tiān　xià　shì.

BE　WHY　SAGACIOUS-　PERSON　EMBRACE　ONE,　FOR　HEAVEN　UNDER　MODEL.

This IS WHY the SAGE EMBRACES the ONE, and serves as a MODEL FOR all things UNDER HEAVEN.

不　自　见，　故　明；

bú　zì　xiàn,　gù　míng;

NOT　SELF　SHOW,　SO　EVIDENT;

He does NOT SHOW HIMSELF, SO he is EVIDENT;

不　自　是，　故　彰；

bú　zì　shì,　gù　zhāng;

NOT　SELF　BE,　SO　ILLUSTRIOUS;

He IS NOT SELF-satisfied, SO he is ILLUSTRIOUS;

不　自　伐，　故　有　功；
bú　zì　fá,　gù　yǒu　gōng;
NOT　SELF　AGGRESSIVE,　SO　HAVE　MERITORIOUS-ACT;
He is NOT AGGRESSIVE, SO he ACCOMPLISHES MERITORIOUS ACTS;

不　自　矜，　故　长。
bú　zì　jīn,　gù　cháng.
NOT　SELF　VAIN,　SO　ADVANTAGE.
He is NOT VAIN, SO he has the ADVANTAGE.

夫　唯　不　争，　故　天　下　莫　能　与
fú　wéi　bù　zhēng,　gù　tiān　xià　mò　néng　yǔ
SINCE　　NOT　CONTEND,　SO　HEAVEN　UNDER　NOT　CAN　WITH

之　争。
zhī　zhēng.
HIM　CONTEND.
SINCE he does NOT CONTEND, NOTHING UNDER HEAVEN CAN CONTEND WITH HIM.

古　之　所　谓　"曲　则　全"　者：
gǔ　zhī　suǒ　wèi　qū　zé　quán　zhě:
ANCIENT　[PART]　[PART]　SAY　CROOKED　YET　WHOLE　[PART]:
The ANCIENT SAYING "CROOKED YET WHOLE:"

岂　虚　言　哉？
qǐ　xū　yán　zāi?
[PART]　EMPTY　WORD　[PART]?
Are these EMPTY WORDS?

诚　全　而　归　之。
chéng　quán　ér　guī　zhī.
INDEED　WHOLE　AND　RETURN　THEM.
INDEED these words are TRUE, AND one can RETURN to THEM.

希　言　自　然。

xī　　yán　　zì　　rán.

LITTLE　TALK　　NATURAL.

It is NATURAL to TALK LITTLE.

故　飘　风　不　终　朝;

gù　　piāo　　fēng　　bù　　zhōng　　zhāo;

FOR　RAGING　WIND　NOT　END　MORNING;

FOR a RAGING WIND does NOT last until the END of the MORNING;

骤　雨　不　终　日。

zhòu　　yǔ　　bù　　zhōng　　rì.

SUDDEN　RAIN　NOT　END　DAY.

A SUDDEN RAIN does NOT last until the END of the DAY.

孰　为　此　者? 天　地。

shú　　wéi　　cǐ　　zhě?　　tiān　　dì.

WHO　CAUSE　THIS　[PART]?　HEAVEN　EARTH.

WHO CAUSES THIS? HEAVEN and EARTH.

天　地　尚　不　能　久,

tiān　　dì　　shàng　　bù　　néng　　jiǔ,

HEAVEN　EARTH　EVEN　NOT　CAN　LONG,

Since EVEN HEAVEN and EARTH CANNOT LONG continue unchanged,

而　况　于　人　乎?

ér　　kuàng　　yú　　rén　　hū?

THEN　HOW　CONCERNING　PERSON　[PART]?

THEN HOW can a PERSON?

故　从　事　于　道　者，同　于　道；
gù　cóng　shì　yú　dào　zhě,　tóng　yú　dào;
FOR　FOLLOW　AFFAIR　WITH　DAO　[PART],　SAME　WITH　DAO;

FOR those WHO FOLLOW the DAO are ONE WITH the DAO;

德　者　同　于　德；
dé　zhě　tóng　yú　dé;
VIRTUE　[PART]　SAME　WITH　VIRTUE;

The VIRTUOUS are ONE WITH VIRTUE;

失　者　同　于　失。
shī　zhě　tóng　yú　shī.
LOSE　[PART]　SAME　WITH　LOSS.

Those WHO LOSE the dao are ONE WITH LOSS.

同　于　道　者，道　亦　乐　得　之；
tóng　yú　dào　zhě,　dào　yì　lè　dé　zhī;
SAME　WITH　DAO　[PART],　DAO　ALSO　GLADLY　GAIN　THEM;

As for those WHO are ONE WITH the DAO, the DAO ALSO GLADLY EXTENDS itself to THEM;

同　于　德　者，德　亦　乐　得　之；
tóng　yú　dé　zhě,　dé　yì　lè　dé　zhī;
SAME　WITH　VIRTUE　[PART],　VIRTUE　ALSO　GLADLY　GAIN　THEM;

As for those WHO are ONE WITH VIRTUE, VIRTUE ALSO GLADLY EXTENDS itself to THEM;

同　于　失　者，失　亦　乐　得　之。
tóng　yú　shī　zhě,　shī　yì　lè　dé　zhī.
SAME　WITH　LOSS　[PART],　LOSS　ALSO　GLADLY　GAIN　THEM.

As for those WHO are ONE WITH LOSS, LOSS ALSO GLADLY EXTENDS itself to THEM.

信　不　足　焉，　有　不　信　焉。

xìn　bù　zú　yān,　yǒu　bú　xìn　yān.

TRUSTWORTHINESS　NOT　SUFFICIENT　[PART],　EXIST　NOT　TRUST　[PART].

If the ruler is NOT SUFFICIENTLY TRUSTWORTHY, there will BE DISTRUST.

企　者　不　立;　跨　者　不　行。

qǐ　zhě　bú　lì;　kuà　zhě　bù　xíng.

TIPTOE　[PART]　NOT　STAND;　STRIDE　[PART]　NOT　WALK.

Those WHO TIPTOE CANNOT STAND firm; those WHO take great STRIDES CANNOT WALK sturdily.

自　见　者　不　明;

zì　xiàn　zhě　bù　míng;

SELF　SHOW　[PART]　NOT　EVIDENT;

Those WHO SHOW THEMSELVES are NOT EVIDENT;

自　是　者　不　彰;

zì　shì　zhě　bù　zhāng;

SELF　BE　[PART]　NOT　ILLUSTRIOUS;

Those WHO ARE SELF-satisfied are NOT ILLUSTRIOUS;

自　伐　者　无　功;

zì　fá　zhě　wú　gōng;

SELF　AGGRESSIVE　[PART]　NOT　MERITORIOUS-ACT;

Those WHO are AGGRESSIVE will accomplish NO MERITORIOUS ACTS;

自　矜　者　不　长。

zì　jīn　zhě　bù　cháng.

SELF　VAIN　[PART]　NOT　ADVANTAGE.

Those WHO are VAIN will NOT have the ADVANTAGE.

其　在　道　也,　日　余　食　赘　形。

qí　zài　dào　yě,　yuē　yú　shí,　zhuì　xíng.

THEY　WITH　DAO　[PART],　CALL　EXCESS　FOOD,　SUPERFLUOUS　FORM.

THOSE who go WITH the DAO CALL these things "EXCESSIVE FOOD" and "SUPERFLUOUS FORM."

物　　或　　恶　　之，

wù　　*huò*　　*wù*　　*zhī,*

MATERIAL　[PART]　LOATHE　THEM,

All the MATERIAL world LOATHES THEM,

故　　有　　道　　者　　不　　处。

gù　　*yǒu*　　*dào*　　*zhě*　　*bù*　　*chǔ.*

SO　　HAVE　　DAO　　[PART]　NOT　　DEAL.

SO those WHO HAVE the DAO do NOT DEAL with them.

有 物 混 成， 先 天 地 生。
yǒu wù hùn chéng, xiān tiān dì shēng.
HAVE SUBSTANCE CHAOS FORM, BEFORE HEAVEN EARTH BORN.

HAVING SUBSTANCE but FORMED from CHAOS, it was BORN BEFORE HEAVEN and EARTH.

寂 兮， 寥 兮， 独 立 而 不 改；
jì xī, liáo xī, dú lì ér bù gǎi;
SILENT [PART], SPARSE [PART], ALONE STAND AND NOT CHANGE;

SILENT and SPARSE, it STANDS ALONE AND NEVER CHANGES;

周 行 而 不 殆；
zhōu xíng ér bú dài;
AROUND GO AND NOT REST;

It is CYCLIC AND NEVER RESTING;

可 以 为 天 地 母。
kě yǐ wéi tiān dì mǔ.
CAN ACT HEAVEN EARTH MOTHER.

It CAN ACT as the MOTHER of HEAVEN and EARTH.

吾 不 知 其 名， 强 字 之 曰 道；
wú bù zhī qí míng, qiáng zì zhī yuē dào;
I NOT KNOW ITS NAME, MUST WORD IT CALL DAO;

I do NOT KNOW ITS NAME, but if I MUST find a WORD for IT, I will CALL it "DAO;"

强 为 之 名 曰 大。
qiáng wèi zhī míng yuē dà.
MUST FOR IT NAME CALL GREAT.

If I MUST find a NAME FOR IT, I will CALL it "GREAT."

大　　　日　　　逝；　　逝　　　日　　　远；　　远　　　日　　　反。

dà　　yuē　　shì;　　shì　　yuē　　yuǎn;　　yuǎn　　yuē　　fǎn.

GREAT　SAY　FLOW;　FLOW　SAY　DISTANT;　DISTANT　SAY　RETURN.

Since it is GREAT, one can SAY that it FLOWS away; since it FLOWS away, one can SAY that it is DISTANT; since it is DISTANT, one can SAY that it will RETURN.

故　　　道　　　大，　天　　　大，　地　　　大，　人　　　亦　　　大。

gù　　dào　　dà,　tiān　　dà,　dì　　dà,　rén　　yì　　dà.

THEREFORE　DAO　GREAT,　HEAVEN　GREAT,　EARTH　GREAT,　MANKIND　ALSO　GREAT.

THEREFORE the DAO is GREAT, HEAVEN is GREAT, the EARTH is GREAT, and MANKIND is ALSO GREAT.

域　　　中　　　有　　　四　　　大，　而　　　人　　　居　　　其　　　一

yù　　zhōng　　yǒu　　sì　　dà,　ér　　rén　　jū　　qí　　yī

UNIVERSE　IN　EXIST　FOUR　GREAT,　AND　MANKIND　BE　THEIR　ONE

焉。

yān.

[PART].

IN the UNIVERSE there ARE FOUR GREAT things, AND MANKIND IS ONE of THEM.

人　　　法　　　地，　地　　　法　　　天，

rén　　fǎ　　dì,　dì　　fǎ　　tiān,

MANKIND　LAW　EARTH,　EARTH　LAW　HEAVEN,

MANKIND takes the EARTH as his LAW, the EARTH takes HEAVEN as its LAW,

天　　　法　　　道，　道　　　法　　　自　　　然。

tiān　　fǎ　　dào,　dào　　fǎ　　zì　　rán.

HEAVEN　LAW　DAO,　DAO　LAW　NATURE.

HEAVEN takes the DAO as its LAW, and the DAO takes NATURE as its LAW.

重　为　轻　根;　静　为　躁　君。
zhòng　wéi　qīng　gēn;　jìng　wéi　zào　jūn.
HEAVY　BE　LIGHT　ROOT;　TRANQUILITY　BE　AGITATION　RULER.

The HEAVY IS the ROOT of the LIGHT; TRANQUILITY IS the RULER of AGITATION.

是　以　君　子　终　日　行　不　离　辎
shì　yǐ　jūn-　zǐ　zhōng　rì　xíng　bù　lí　zī
BE　WHY　NOBLE-　PERSON　END　DAY　TRAVEL　NOT　LEAVE　SUPPLY-

重。
zhòng.
CART.

This IS WHY the NOBLE PERSON, TRAVELING to the END of the DAY, does NOT STRAY from the military EQUIPMENT.

虽　有　荣　观,　燕　处　超　然。
suī　yǒu　róng　guān,　yàn　chù　chāo　rán.
THOUGH　EXIST　EXQUISITE　SIGHT,　SWALLOW　PLACE,　PASS　[PART].

THOUGH there ARE EXQUISITE SIGHTS and PLACES where SWALLOWS fly, he PASSES them by.

奈　何　万　乘　之　主,
nài　hé　wàn　shèng　zhī　zhǔ,
HOW　　TEN-THOUSAND　CHARIOT　[PART]　MASTER,

HOW can one be MASTER OF TEN THOUSAND CHARIOTS,

而　以　身　轻　天　下?
ér　yǐ　shēn　qīng　tiān　xià?
BUT　TAKE　BODY　LIGHTLY　HEAVEN　UNDER?

BUT ACT LIGHTLY UNDER HEAVEN?

轻　则　失　根;　躁　则　失　君。
qīng　zé　shī　gēn;　zào　zé　shī　jūn.
LIGHT　SO　LOSE　ROOT;　AGITATED　SO　LOSE　SOVEREIGN.

Those who act LIGHTLY will LOSE the ROOT; those who are AGITATED will LOSE CONTROL.

善　行，无　辙　迹；
shàn　*xíng,*　*wú*　*zhé-*　*jì;*
GOOD　WALK,　NOT　TRACK-　TRACE;

Those who are GOOD at WALKING leave NO TRACKS;

善　言，无　瑕　谪；
shàn　*yán,*　*wú*　*xiá-*　*zhé;*
GOOD　SPEAK,　NOT　FLAW-　BLAME;

Those who are GOOD at SPEAKING make NO ERRORS;

善　数，不　用　筹　策；
shàn　*shǔ,*　*bú*　*yòng*　*chóu-*　*cè;*
GOOD　CALCULATE,　NOT　USE　COUNTING-　CHIP;

Those who are GOOD at CALCULATING USE NO COUNTING CHIPS;

善　闭，无　关　楗　而　不　可　开；
shàn　*bì,*　*wú*　*guān-*　*jiàn*　*ér*　*bù*　*kě*　*kāi;*
GOOD　CLOSE　NOT　LOCK-　KEY　YET　NOT　CAN　OPEN;

Those who are GOOD at CLOSING things use NO KEY, YET what they close CANNOT be OPENED;

善　结，无　绳　约　而　不　可　解。
shàn　*jié,*　*wú*　*shéng*　*yuē*　*ér*　*bù*　*kě*　*jiě.*
GOOD　TIE,　NOT　ROPE　BIND　YET　NOT　CAN　UNTIE.

Those who are GOOD at TYING use NO ROPE for BINDING, YET what they tie CANNOT be UNTIED.

是　以　圣　人　常　善　救　人；
shì　*yǐ*　*shèng-*　*rén*　*cháng*　*shàn*　*jiù*　*rén;*
BE　WHY　SAGACIOUS-　PERSON　ALWAYS　GOOD　HELP　PEOPLE;

This IS WHY the SAGE is ALWAYS GOOD at HELPING PEOPLE;

故　无　弃　人;
gù　wú　qì　rén;
SO　NOT　ABANDON　PERSON;
He ABANDONS NO ONE;

常　善　救　物,　故　无　弃　物。
cháng　shàn　jiù　wù,　gù　wú　qì　wù.
ALWAYS　GOOD　SAVE　THING,　SO　NOT　ABANDON　THING.
He is ALWAYS GOOD at CARING for THINGS, SO he ABANDONS NOTHING.

是　谓　袭　明。
shì　wèi　xí　míng.
BE　CALL　PERPETUATE　BRIGHT.
This IS CALLED "PERPETUATING BRIGHTNESS."

故　善　人　者,　不　善　人　之　师。
gù　shàn　rén　zhě,　bú　shàn　rén　zhī　shī.
THEREFORE　GOOD　PERSON　[PART],　NOT　GOOD　PERSON　[PART]　TEACHER.
THEREFORE the GOOD PERSON is the TEACHER OF THOSE who are NOT GOOD.

不　善　人　者,　善　人　之　资。
bú　shàn　rén　zhě,　shàn　rén　zhī　zī.
NOT　GOOD　PERSON　[PART],　GOOD　PERSON　[PART]　CAPITAL.
THOSE WHO are NOT GOOD are the STUDENTS OF the GOOD PERSON.

不　贵　其　师,　不　爱　其　资,
bú　guì　qí　shī,　bú　ài　qí　zī,
NOT　ESTEEM　ONE'S　TEACHER,　NOT　LOVE　ONE'S　CAPITAL,
If one does NOT ESTEEM ONE'S TEACHER, if one does NOT LOVE ONE'S STUDENTS,

虽　智　大　迷。

suī　　*zhì*　　*dà*　　*mí.*

ALTHOUGH　INTELLECT　GREAT　CONFUSION.

ALTHOUGH there may be INTELLECT, there will be GREAT CONFUSION.

是　谓　要　妙。

shì　　*wèi*　　*yào*　　*miào.*

BE　　CALL　　DEEP　　MYSTERY.

This IS CALLED "a DEEP MYSTERY."

知　　其　　雄，　守　　其　　雌；

zhī   *qí*   *xióng,*   *shǒu*   *qí*   *cí;*
KNOW   ITS   MASCULINE,   PRESERVE   ITS   FEMININE;

KNOW the MASCULINE but PRESERVE the FEMININE;

为　　天　　下　　溪。

wéi   *tiān*   *xià*   *xī.*
SERVE   HEAVEN   UNDER   WATERCOURSE.

SERVE as a WATERCOURSE for all things UNDER HEAVEN.

为　　天　　下　　溪，　常　　德　　不　　离；

wéi   *tiān*   *xià*   *xī,*   *cháng*   *dé*   *bù*   *lí;*
SERVE   HEAVEN   UNDER   WATERCOURSE,   UNCHANGING   VIRTUE   NOT   LEAVE;

SERVING as a WATERCOURSE for all things UNDER HEAVEN, do NOT LEAVE the UNCHANGING VIRTUE;

复　　归　　于　　婴　　儿。

fù-   *guī*   *yú*   *yīng-*   *ér.*
TURN-   RETURN   TO   BABY-   CHILD.

RETURN TO the nature of a BABY.

知　　其　　白，　守　　其　　黑；

zhī   *qí*   *bái,*   *shǒu*   *qí*   *hēi;*
KNOWS   ITS   WHITE,   PRESERVE   ITS   BLACK;

KNOW WHITENESS but PRESERVE BLACKNESS;

为　　天　　下　　式。

wéi   *tiān*   *xià*   *shì.*
SERVE   HEAVEN   UNDER   MODEL.

SERVE as a MODEL for all things UNDER HEAVEN.

为　天　下　式，常　德　不　忒；

wéi　tiān　xià　shì,　cháng　dé　bú　tè;

SERVE　HEAVEN　UNDER　MODEL,　UNCHANGING　VIRTUE　NOT　FAULT;

SERVING as a MODEL for all things UNDER HEAVEN, carry out the UNCHANGING VIRTUE WITHOUT FAULT;

复　归　于　无　极。

fù-　guī　yú　wú　jí.

TURN-　RETURN　TO　NOT　LIMIT.

RETURN TO the INFINITE.

知　其　荣，守　其　辱；

zhī　qí　róng,　shǒu　qí　rǔ;

KNOW　ITS　HONOR,　PRESERVE　ITS　DISGRACE;

KNOW HONOR but PRESERVE DISGRACE;

为　天　下　谷。

wéi　tiān　xià　gǔ.

SERVE　HEAVEN　UNDER　VALLEY.

SERVE as a VALLEY for all things UNDER HEAVEN.

为　天　下　谷，常　德　乃　足；

wéi　tiān　xià　gǔ,　cháng　dé　nǎi　zú;

SERVE　HEAVEN　UNDER　VALLEY,　UNCHANGING　VIRTUE　BE　COMPLETE;

SERVING as a VALLEY for all things UNDER HEAVEN, allow the UNCHANGING VIRTUE to BE COMPLETE;

复　归　于　朴。

fù-　guī　yú　pǔ.

TURN-　RETURN　TO　BLOCK-OF-WOOD.

RETURN TO the nature of a BLOCK OF WOOD.

朴　散，　则　为　器。
pǔ　*sàn,*　*zé*　*wéi*　*qì.*
BLOCK-OF-WOOD BREAK-UP,　BUT　SERVE-AS　IMPLEMENT.
The BLOCK OF WOOD can be CARVED, BUT then it will SERVE AS an IMPLEMENT.

圣　人　用　之，　则　为　官　长。
shèng-　*rén*　*yòng*　*zhī,*　*zé*　*wéi*　*guān-*　*zhǎng.*
SAGACIOUS-　PERSON　USE　IT,　AND　SERVE-AS　OFFICER-　LEADER.
The SAGE USES IT AND SERVES AS RULER.

故　大　制　不　割。
gù　*dà*　*zhì*　*bù*　*gē.*
THEREFORE　GREAT　CRAFT　NOT　CUT.
THEREFORE the GREAT CRAFTSMAN does NOT CUT.

Chapter 29

将 欲 取 天 下 而 为 之,

jiāng   *yù*   *qǔ*   *tiān*   *xià*   *ér*   *wéi*   *zhī,*

FUTURE   DESIRE   TAKE   HEAVEN   UNDER   AND   ACT   THEM,

If one DESIRES to RULE all things UNDER HEAVEN AND ACT on THEM,

吾 见 其 不 得 已。

wú   *jiàn*   *qí*   *bù*   *dé*   *yǐ.*

I   REGARD   IT   NOT   GAIN   [PART].

I REGARD THIS as UNACHIEVABLE.

天 下 神 器:

tiān   *xià*   *shén*   *qì:*

HEAVEN   UNDER   SACRED   IMPLEMENT:

The UNIVERSE is a SACRED IMPLEMENT:

不 可 为 也; 不 可 执 也。

bù   *kě*   *wéi*   *yě;*   *bù*   *kě*   *zhí*   *yě.*

NOT   CAN   ACT   [PART];   NOT   CAN   HOLD   [PART].

One CANNOT ACT on it; one CANNOT HOLD it.

为 者 败 之; 执 者 失 之。

wéi   *zhě*   *bài*   *zhī;*   *zhí*   *zhě*   *shī*   *zhī.*

ACT   [PART]   RUIN   IT;   HOLD   [PART]   LOSE   IT.

Those WHO ACT on it RUIN IT; those who HOLD it LOSE IT.

是 以 圣 人 无 为。

shì   *yǐ*   *shèng-*   *rén*   *wú*   *wéi.*

BE   WHY   SAGACIOUS-   PERSON   NOT   ACT.

This IS WHY the SAGE does NOT ACT.

故 无 败; 故 无 失。

gù   *wú*   *bài;*   *gù*   *wú*   *shī.*

THEREFORE   NOT   RUIN;   THEREFORE   NOT   LOSE.

THEREFORE he does NOT RUIN it; THEREFORE he does NOT LOSE it.

夫	物	或	行	或	随;	或	觑	或	吹;
fú	wù	huò	xíng	huò	suí;	huò	xū	huò	chuī;
FOR	THING	EITHER	GO	OR	FOLLOW;	EITHER	SIGH	OR	BLOW;

FOR THINGS EITHER GO before OR FOLLOW; one EITHER SIGHS lightly or BREATHES hard;

或	强	或	羸;	或	载	或	隳。
huò	qiáng	huò	léi;	huò	zài	huò	huī.
EITHER	STRONG	OR	WEAK;	EITHER	CARRY	OR	DESTROY.

Things are EITHER STRONG OR WEAK; they EITHER FUNCTION OR are DESTROYED.

是	以	圣	人	去	甚,	去	奢,	去	泰。
shì	yǐ	shèng-	rén	qù	shèn,	qù	shē,	qù	tài.
BE	WHY	SAGACIOUS-	PERSON	GO	EXTREME,	GO	LUXURY,	GO	EXCESS.

This IS WHY the SAGE LEAVES EXTREMES, LUXURY, and EXCESS.

Chapter 30

以　道　佐　人　主　者，
yǐ　dào　zuǒ　rén-　zhǔ　zhě,
USE　DAO　ASSIST　PERSON-　RULE　[PART],

Those WHO USE the DAO to ASSIST the RULER

不　以　兵　强　天　下。
bù　yǐ　bīng　qiáng　tiān　xià.
NOT　USE　MILITARY　FORCE　HEAVEN　UNDER.

Do NOT USE MILITARY might to FORCE all things UNDER HEAVEN.

其　事　好　还。
qí　shì　hào　huán.
ITS　ACT　LIKELY　RETRIBUTION.

MILITARY ACTS are LIKELY to provoke RETRIBUTION.

师　之　所　处，荆　棘　生　焉。
shī　zhī　suǒ　chǔ,　jīng　jí　shēng　yān.
ARMY　[PART]　WHERE　LOCATE,　THISTLES　THORNS　GROW　[PART].

WHEREVER the ARMY has BEEN, THISTLES and THORNS are GROWING.

大　军　之　后，必　有　凶　年。
dà　jūn　zhī　hòu,　bì　yǒu　xiōng　nián.
GREAT　BATTLE　[PART]　AFTER,　MUST　EXIST　SEVERE　YEAR.

AFTER a GREAT BATTLE, there MUST FOLLOW YEARS of FAMINE.

善　有　果　而　已; 不　敢　以　取　强;
shàn　yǒu　guǒ　ér　yǐ;　bù　gǎn　yǐ　qǔ　qiáng.
BENEVOLENTLY　HAVE　SUCCESS　[PART];　NOT　DARE　USE　TAKE　FORCE.

One should HANDLE SUCCESS BENEVOLENTLY; one should NOT DARE USE it to TAKE things and FORCE them.

果　而　勿　矜；果　而　勿　伐；

guǒ　　ér　　wù　　jīn;　　guǒ　　ér　　wù　　fá;
SUCCESS　BUT　NOT　VAIN;　SUCCESS　BUT　NOT　AGGRESSIVE;

Achieve SUCCESS, BUT WITHOUT VANITY; achieve SUCCESS, BUT WITHOUT AGGRESSION;

果　而　勿　骄；果　而　不　得　已；

guǒ　　ér　　wù　　jiāo;　　guǒ　　ér　　bù　　dé　　yǐ;
SUCCESS　BUT　NOT　ARROGANT;　SUCCESS　BUT　NOT　GAIN　[PART];

Achieve SUCCESS, BUT WITHOUT ARROGANCE; achieve SUCCESS, BUT WITHOUT GAIN;

果　而　勿　强。

guǒ　　ér　　wù　　qiáng.
SUCCESS　BUT　NOT　FORCE.

Achieve SUCCESS, BUT WITHOUT FORCE.

物　壮　则　老。

wù　　zhuàng　　zé　　lǎo.
THING　STRONG　BUT　OLD.

THINGS may be STRONG, BUT they will become OLD and weak.

是　谓　不　道；不　道　早　已。

shì　　wèi　　bú　　dào;　　bú　　dào　　zǎo　　yǐ.
BE　SAY　NOT　DAO;　NOT　DAO　EARLY　END.

It IS SAID that this is NOT the DAO; all things NOT with the DAO meet an EARLY END.

夫　兵　者，　不　祥　之　器。

fú　bīng　zhě,　bù　xiáng　zhī　qì.
FOR　WEAPON　[PART]　NOT　AUSPICIOUS　[PART]　IMPLEMENT.

FOR WEAPONS are INAUSPICIOUS IMPLEMENTS.

物　或　恶　之，

wù　huò　wù　zhī,
MATERIAL　[PART]　LOATHE　THEM,

All the MATERIAL world LOATHES THEM,

故　有　道　者　不　处。

gù　yǒu　dào　zhě　bù　chǔ.
SO　HAVE　DAO　[PART]·　NOT　DEAL.

SO those WHO HAVE the DAO do NOT DEAL with weapons.

君　子　居，　则　贵　左，

jūn-　zǐ　jū,　zé　guì　zuǒ,
NOBLE-　PERSON　RESIDE,　AND　EMPHASIZE　LEFT,

When the NOBLE PERSON RESIDES at home he EMPHASIZES the LEFT,

用　兵，　则　贵　右。

yòng　bīng,　zé　guì　yòu.
USE　WEAPON,　BUT　EMPHASIZE　RIGHT.

BUT when he USES WEAPONS he EMPHASIZES the RIGHT.

兵　者　不　祥　之　器，

bīng　zhě　bù　xiáng　zhī　qì,
WEAPON　[PART]　NOT　AUSPICIOUS　[PART]　IMPLEMENT,

WEAPONS are INAUSPICIOUS IMPLEMENTS,

非　君　子　之　器。

fēi   jūn-   zǐ   zhī   qì.
NOT   NOBLE- PERSON [PART] IMPLEMENT.

NOT the IMPLEMENTS OF the NOBLE PERSON.

不　得　已　而　用　之。

bù   dé   yǐ   ér   yòng   zhī.
NOT   GAIN END   AND   USE   THEM.

Only when he HAS NO CHOICE does he USE THEM.

恬　淡　为　上;　胜　而　不　美。

tián   dàn   wéi   shàng;   shèng   ér   bù   měi.
QUIET CALM   BE   SUPERIOR; VICTORY AND   NOT BEAUTIFUL.

QUIET and CALM ARE BEST; one can gain VICTORY AND NOT consider it BEAUTIFUL.

而　美　之　者,　是　乐　杀　人。

ér   měi   zhī   zhě,   shì   lè   shā   rén.
BUT BEAUTIFUL IT   [PART], BE   EXULT KILL PERSON.

BUT those WHO consider IT BEAUTIFUL ARE EXULTING in KILLING.

夫　乐　杀　人　者,

fú   lè   shā   rén   zhě,
FOR   EXULT KILL PERSON [PART],

FOR those WHO EXULT in KILLING

则　不　可　以　得　志　于　天　下　矣。

zé   bù   kě   yǐ   dé   zhì   yú   tiān   xià   yǐ.
SO   NOT   CAN   ACHIEVE ASPIRATION IN HEAVEN UNDER [PART].

CANNOT ACHIEVE their ASPIRATIONS IN the UNIVERSE.

吉　事　尚　左；　凶　事　尚　右。

jí　　　shì　　shàng　zuǒ;　　xiōng　shì　　shàng　yòu.
AUSPICIOUS EVENT　VALUE　LEFT;　SEVERE　EVENT　VALUE　RIGHT.

In AUSPICIOUS TIMES, VALUE is placed on the LEFT; in SEVERE TIMES, VALUE is placed on the RIGHT.

偏　将　军　居　左；　上　将　军　居　右。

piān　jiāng-　jūn　jū　　zuǒ;　shàng　jiāng-　jūn　　jū　　yòu.
SIDE　ARMY-　RULER　OCCUPY　LEFT;　CHIEF　ARMY-　RULER　OCCUPY　RIGHT.

The GENERAL OCCUPIES the LEFT; the CHIEF MARTIAL OCCUPIES the RIGHT.

言　以　丧　礼　处　之。

yán　yǐ　　sāng　lǐ　　chǔ　zhī.
SAY　TAKE　FUNERAL　RITE　DEAL　THEM.

It is SAID that one should CONDUCT a FUNERAL RITE to DEAL with the SLAIN.

杀　人　之　众，　以　悲　哀　泣　之；

shā　rén　zhī　zhòng,　yǐ　　bēi　　āi　　lì　　zhī;
SLAIN　PERSON　[PART]　NUMEROUS,　[PART]　SORROWFUL　MOURNING　GO　THEM;

As for the MULTITUDE OF the SLAIN, one should GO to THEM WITH SORROWFUL MOURNING;

战　胜　以　丧　礼　处　之。

zhàn　shèng　yǐ　　sāng　lǐ　　chǔ　zhī
BATTLE　WIN　TAKE　FUNERAL　RITE　DEAL　THEM.

When the BATTLE is WON, one should CONDUCT a FUNERAL RITE to DEAL with the SLAIN.

道　常　无　名；朴　虽　小，

dào　cháng　wú　míng;　pǔ　suī　xiǎo,

DAO　UNCHANGINGLY　NOT　NAME;　SIMPLE　ALTHOUGH　SMALL,

The DAO is UNCHANGINGLY NAMELESS; ALTHOUGH it is SIMPLE and SMALL,

天　下　莫　能　臣。

tiān　xià　mò　néng　chén.

UNDER　HEAVEN　NOT　CAN　CONTROL.

UNDER HEAVEN there is NOTHING that CAN CONTROL it.

侯　王　若　能　守　之，

hóu　wáng　ruò　néng　shǒu　zhī,

PRINCE　KING　IF　CAN　PRESERVE　IT,

IF PRINCES and KINGS CAN PRESERVE IT,

万　物　将　自　宾。

wàn　wù　jiāng　zì　bīn.

TEN-THOUSAND　THING　WILL　SELF　OBEY.

ALL THINGS WILL WILLINGLY OBEY.

天　地　相　合，以　降　甘　露。

tiān　dì　xiāng　hé,　yǐ　jiàng　gān　lù.

HEAVEN　EARTH　MUTUALLY　UNITE,　[PART]　FALL　SWEET　DEW.

HEAVEN and EARTH will MUTUALLY UNITE, and CAUSE the SWEET DEW to FALL.

民　莫　之　令　而　自　匀。

mín　mò　zhī　lìng　ér　zì　yún.

PEOPLE　NOT　THEM　COMMAND　BUT　SELF　BALANCE.

As for the PEOPLE, there will be NO ONE COMMANDING THEM, BUT they will achieve BALANCE by THEMSELVES.

始　制　有　名。名　亦　既　有，
shǐ　zhì　yǒu　míng.　míng　yì　jì　yǒu,
BEGIN　CONTROL　HAVE　RENOWN.　RENOWN　EVEN　IF　HAVE,

Those who have ESTABLISHED CONTROL HAVE RENOWN. But EVEN IF one HAS RENOWN,

夫　亦　将　知　止；知　止　可　以　不
fú　yì　jiāng　zhī　zhǐ;　zhī　zhǐ　kě　yǐ　bú
SO　ALSO　FUTURE　KNOW　STOP;　KNOW　STOP　CAN　　NOT

殆。
dài.
HARM.

One MUST ALSO KNOW when to STOP; if one KNOWS when to STOP, one CAN AVOID HARM.

譬　道　之　在　天　下，
pì　dào　zhī　zài　tiān　xià,
FOR　DAO　GO　IN　HEAVEN　UNDER,

FOR the DAO GOES THROUGH the UNIVERSE

犹　川　谷　之　于　江　海。
yóu　chuān　gǔ　zhī　yú　jiāng　hǎi.
LIKE　RIVER　VALLEY　GO　TO　RIVER　OCEAN.

LIKE a RIVER VALLEY LEADING TO RIVERS and OCEANS.

知　人　者　智；自　知　者　明。

zhī 　 *rén* 　 *zhě* 　 *zhì;* 　 *zì* 　 *zhī* 　 *zhě* 　 *míng.*
KNOW 　 PERSON 　 [PART] 　 WISDOM; 　 SELF 　 KNOW 　 [PART] 　 ENLIGHTENED.

Those WHO KNOW OTHERS have WISDOM; those WHO KNOW THEMSELVES are ENLIGHTENED.

胜　人　者　有　力，自　胜　者　强。

shèng 　 *rén* 　 *zhě* 　 *yǒu* 　 *lì,* 　 *zì* 　 *shèng* 　 *zhě* 　 *qiáng.*
CONQUER 　 PERSON 　 [PART] 　 HAVE 　 POWER, 　 SELF 　 CONQUER 　 [PART] 　 STRONG.

Those WHO CONQUER OTHERS HAVE POWER, but those WHO CONQUER THEMSELVES have inner STRENGTH.

知　足　者　富。

zì 　 *zú* 　 *zhě* 　 *fù.*
KNOW 　 ENOUGH 　 [PART] 　 RICH.

Those WHO KNOW when they have ENOUGH are RICH.

强　行　者　有　志。

qiáng 　 *xíng* 　 *zhě* 　 *yǒu* 　 *zhì.*
STRONGLY 　 PROCEED 　 [PART] 　 HAVE 　 WILL.

Those WHO PROCEED RESOLUTELY HAVE great force of WILL.

不　失　其　所　者　久。

bù 　 *shī* 　 *qí* 　 *suǒ* 　 *zhě* 　 *jiǔ.*
NOT 　 LOSE 　 THEY 　 POSSESS 　 [PART] 　 LONG.

Those WHO do NOT LOSE what THEY POSSESS will LONG continue.

死　而　不　亡　者　寿。

sǐ 　 *ér* 　 *bù* 　 *wáng* 　 *zhě* 　 *shòu.*
DIE 　 BUT 　 NOT 　 PERISH 　 [PART] 　 LONGEVITY.

Those WHO DIE BUT do NOT PERISH possess LONGEVITY.

Chapter 34

大　道　汜　兮；其　可　左　右。
dà　dào　sì　xī;　qí　kě　zuǒ　yòu.
GREAT　DAO　FLOOD　[PART];　IT　CAN　LEFT　RIGHT.

The GREAT DAO is a FLOOD; IT CAN flow LEFT or RIGHT.

万　物　恃　之　以　生　而　不　辞。
wàn　wù　shì　zhī　yǐ　shēng　ér　bù　cí.
TEN-THOUSAND　THING　DEPEND　IT　TO　LIVE　AND　NOT　DEPART.

ALL THINGS DEPEND on IT TO LIVE, AND it NEVER DEPARTS.

功　成　而　不　有。
gōng　chéng　ér　bù　yǒu.
MERITORIOUS-ACT　ACCOMPLISH　BUT　NOT　POSSESS.

It ACCOMPLISHES MERITORIOUS ACTS, BUT does NOT POSSESS.

衣　养　万　物　而　不　为　主；
yī　yǎng　wàn　wù　ér　bù　wéi　zhǔ;
CLOTHE　CARE　TEN-THOUSAND　THING　BUT　NOT　ACT　MASTER;

It CLOTHES and CARES for ALL THINGS, BUT does NOT ACT as their MASTER;

可　名　于　小。
kě　míng　yú　xiǎo.
CAN　CALL　AS　SMALL.

It CAN be CALLED "SMALL."

万　物　归　焉　而　不　为　主；
wàn　wù　guī　yān　ér　bù　wéi　zhǔ;
TEN-THOUSAND　THING　RETURN　[PART]　BUT　NOT　ACT　MASTER;

ALL THINGS RETURN to it, BUT it does NOT ACT as their MASTER;

可　名　为　大。

kě　*míng*　*wéi*　*dà.*
CAN　CALL　AS　GREAT.

It CAN be CALLED "GREAT."

以　其　终　不　自　为　大，

yǐ　*qí*　*zhōng*　*bú*　*zì*　*wéi*　*dà,*
SINCE　IT　END　NOT　SELF　ACT　GREAT,

SINCE in the END it does NOT INTENTIONALLY ACT GREAT,

故　能　成　其　大。

gù　*néng*　*chéng*　*qí*　*dà.*
THEREFORE　ABLE　ACHIEVE　ITS　GREAT.

It is ABLE to ACHIEVE ITS GREATNESS.

Chapter 35

执 大 象, 天 下 往。

zhí   dà   xiàng,   tiān   xià   wǎng.
HOLD   GREAT   IMAGE,   HEAVEN   UNDER   GO.

As for the one who HOLDS to the GREAT IMAGE of the dao, all things UNDER HEAVEN GO to him.

往 而 不 害, 安 平 太。

wǎng   ér   bú   hài,   ān   píng   tài.
GO   BUT   NOT   HARM,   SO   CALM   PEACE.

They GO to him BUT do NO HARM, SO there is CALM and PEACE.

乐 与 饵; 过 客 止。

yuè   yǔ   ěr;   guò   kè   zhǐ.
MUSIC   AND   FOOD;   PASS   GUEST   STOP.

There are MUSIC AND REFRESHMENT; PASSING GUESTS STOP.

道 之 出 口, 淡 乎; 其 无 味。

dào   zhī   chū   kǒu,   dàn   hū;   qí   wú   wèi.
DAO   [PART]   LEAVE   MOUTH,   TASTELESS   [PART];   IT   NO   FLAVOR.

When the word "DAO" LEAVES the MOUTH, it is TASTELESS; IT has NO FLAVOR.

视 之 不 足 见;

shì   zhī   bù   zú   jiàn;
WATCH   IT   NOT   ENOUGH   SEE;

If one WATCHES for IT, there is NOT ENOUGH to be SEEN;

听 之 不 足 闻;

tīng   zhī   bù   zú   wén;
LISTEN   IT   NOT   ENOUGH   HEAR;

If one LISTENS for IT, there is NOT ENOUGH to be HEARD;

用 之 不 足 既。

yòng   zhī   bù   zú   jì.
USE   IT   NOT   ENOUGH   CONSUME.

If one USES IT, there is NOT ENOUGH to be CONSUMED.

将　欲　歙　之，必　固　张　之。

jiāng　*yù*　*xī*　*zhī,*　*bì*　*gù*　*zhāng*　*zhī.*
FUTURE　DESIRE　RESTRAIN　IT,　　MUST　　EXPAND　IT.

IF one DESIRES to RESTRAIN IT, one MUST EXPAND IT.

将　欲　弱　之，必　固　强　之。

jiāng　*yù*　*ruò*　*zhī,*　*bì*　*gù*　*qiáng*　*zhī.*
FUTURE　DESIRE　WEAKEN　IT,　　MUST　STRENGTHEN　IT.

IF one DESIRES to WEAKEN IT, one MUST STRENGTHEN IT.

将　欲　废　之，必　固　兴　之。

jiāng　*yù*　*fèi*　*zhī,*　*bì*　*gù*　*xīng*　*zhī.*
FUTURE　DESIRE　ABOLISH　IT,　　MUST　PROMOTE　IT.

IF one DESIRES to ABOLISH IT, one MUST PROMOTE IT.

将　欲　取　之，必　固　与　之。

jiāng　*yù*　*qǔ*　*zhī,*　*bì*　*gù*　*yǔ*　*zhī.*
FUTURE　DESIRE　TAKE　IT,　　MUST　GIVE　IT.

IF one DESIRES to TAKE IT, one MUST GIVE IT.

是　谓　微　明。

shì　*wèi*　*wēi*　*míng.*
BE　CALL　PROFOUND UNDERSTANDING.

This IS CALLED "PROFOUND UNDERSTANDING."

柔　弱　胜　刚　强。

róu　*ruò*　*shèng*　*gāng*　*qiáng.*
SOFT　WEAK　CONQUER　FIRM　STRONG.

The SOFT and WEAK CONQUERS the FIRM and STRONG.

鱼　不　可　脱　于　渊；

yú　　bù　　kě　　tuō　　yú　　yuān;

FISH　　NOT　　CAN　　TAKE　　FROM　　POOL;

A FISH CANNOT be TAKEN FROM its POOL;

国　之　利　器　不　可　以　示　人。

guó　　zhī　　lì　　qì　　bù　　kě　　yǐ　　shì　　rén.

COUNTRY　[PART]　SHARP　IMPLEMENT　NOT　　CAN　　　SHOW　PERSON.

A COUNTRY'S WEAPONS SHOULD be SHOWN to NO ONE.

道　常　无　为　而　无　不　为。

dào　cháng　wú　wéi　ér　wú　bù　wéi.

DAO　UNCHANGINGLY　NOT　ACT　BUT　NOT　NOT　ACT.

The DAO is UNCHANGINGLY NON-ACTING, BUT there is NOTHING that it does NOT ACHIEVE.

侯　王　若　能　守　之，

hóu　wáng　ruò　néng　shǒu　zhī,

PRINCE　KING　IF　CAN　PRESERVE　IT,

IF PRINCES and KINGS CAN PRESERVE IT,

万　物　将　自　化。

wàn　wù　jiāng　zì　huà.

TEN-THOUSAND THING　WILL　SELF　TRANSFORM.

ALL THINGS WILL TRANSFORM THEMSELVES.

化　而　欲　作，

huà　ér　yù　zuò,

TRANSFORM　AND　DESIRE　DEVELOP,

If they TRANSFORM themselves AND DESIRES DEVELOP,

吾　将　镇　之　以　无　名　之　朴。

wú　jiāng　zhèn　zhī　yǐ　wú　míng　zhī　pǔ.

I　WILL　COOL　THEM　USE　NOT　NAME　[PART]　SIMPLE.

I WILL COOL THEM USING the SIMPLICITY OF the UNNAMED.

镇　之　以　无　名　之　朴，夫　将　不

zhèn　zhī　yǐ　wú　míng　zhī　pǔ,　fú　jiāng　bú

COOL　THEM　USE　NOT　NAME　[PART]　SIMPLE,　SO　WILL　NOT

欲。

yù.

DESIRE.

If I COOL THEM USING the SIMPLICITY OF the UNNAMED, there WILL be NO DESIRES.

不　欲　以　静，天　下　将　自　定。

bú　　yù　　yǐ　　jìng,　　tiān　　xià　　jiāng　　zì　　dìng.

NOT　DESIRE　TAKE　TRANQUIL,　HEAVEN　UNDER　WILL　SELF　CALM.

If there are NO DESIRES there will BE TRANQUILITY, so all things UNDER HEAVEN WILL CALM THEMSELVES.

上　德　不　德；是　以　有　德；

shàng　dé　bù　dé;　shì　yǐ　yǒu　dé;

SUPERIOR　VIRTUE　NOT　VIRTUE;　BE　WHY　HAVE　VIRTUE;

SUPERIOR VIRTUE is NOT superficial VIRTUE; this IS WHY it HAS VIRTUE;

下　德　不　失　德；是　以　无　德。

xià　dé　bù　shī　dé;　shì　yǐ　wú　dé.

INFERIOR　VIRTUE　NOT　LOSE　VIRTUE;　BE　WHY　NOT　VIRTUE.

INFERIOR VIRTUE NEVER LOSES superficial VIRTUE; this IS WHY it is NOT VIRTUE.

上　德　无　为　而　无　以　为；

shàng　dé　wú　wéi　ér　wú　yǐ　wéi;

SUPERIOR　VIRTUE　NOT　ACT　BUT　NOT　TAKE　ACT;

SUPERIOR VIRTUE does NOT ACT, BUT this occurs WITHOUT INTENT;

下　德　无　为　而　有　以　为。

xià　dé　wú　wéi　ér　yǒu　yǐ　wéi.

INFERIOR　VIRTUE　NOT　ACT　BUT　HAVE　TAKE　ACT.

INFERIOR VIRTUE does NOT ACT, BUT this OCCURS INTENTIONALLY.

上　仁　为　之　而　无　以　为；

shàng　rén　wéi　zhī　ér　wú　yǐ　wéi;

SUPERIOR BENEVOLENCE　ACT　IT　BUT　NOT　TAKE　ACT;

SUPERIOR BENEVOLENCE ACTS, BUT this occurs WITHOUT INTENT;

上　义　为　之　而　有　以　为。

shàng　yì　wéi　zhī　ér　yǒu　yǐ　wéi.

SUPERIOR RIGHTEOUSNESS　ACT　IT　BUT　HAVE　TAKE　ACT.

SUPERIOR RIGHTEOUSNESS ACTS, BUT this OCCURS INTENTIONALLY.

上　礼　为　之　而　莫　之　应，

shàng　lǐ　wéi　zhī　ér　mò　zhī　yìng,

SUPERIOR　RITUAL　ACT　IT　BUT　NOT　ITS　RESPONSE,

If SUPERIOR RITUAL ACTS, BUT there is NO RESPONSE,

则　　攘　　臂　　而　　扔　　之。
zé　　răng　　bì　　ér　　rēng　　zhī.
THEN　　BARE　　ARM　　AND　　THROW　　THEM.
THEN it BARES its ARMS and FORCES THINGS.

故　　失　　道　　而　　后　　德;
gù　　shī　　dào　　ér　　hòu　　dé;
THEREFORE　　LOSE　　DAO　　[PART]　　AFTER　　VIRTUE;
THEREFORE AFTER the DAO is LOST, VIRTUE remains;

失　　德　　而　　后　　仁;
shī　　dé　　ér　　hòu　　rén;
LOSE　　VIRTUE　　[PART]　　AFTER　　BENEVOLENCE;
AFTER VIRTUE is LOST, BENEVOLENCE remains;

失　　仁　　而　　后　　义;
shī　　rén　　ér　　hòu　　yì;
LOSE　　BENEVOLENCE　　[PART]　　AFTER　　RIGHTEOUSNESS;
AFTER BENEVOLENCE is LOST, RIGHTEOUSNESS remains;

失　　义　　而　　后　　礼。
shī　　yì　　ér　　hòu　　lǐ.
LOSE　　RIGHTEOUSNESS　　[PART]　　AFTER　　RITUAL.
AFTER RIGHTEOUSNESS is LOST, RITUAL REMAINS.

夫　　礼　　者,　　忠　　信　　之　　薄,
fú　　lǐ　　zhě,　　zhōng　　xìn　　zhī　　bó,
FOR　　RITUAL　　[PART],　　LOYAL　　TRUST　　[PART]　　THIN,
FOR those WHO emphasize RITUAL bring with them THIN LOYALTIES

而　　乱　　之　　首;
ér　　luàn　　zhī　　shǒu;
AND　　DISORDER　　[PART]　　BEGINNING;
AND the BEGINNING OF DISORDER;

前 识 者, 道 之 华,

qián   *shí*   *zhě,*   *dào*   *zhī*   *huá,*
BEFORE   KNOW   [PART],   DAO   [PART]   FLASHY,

SOOTHSAYERS reduce the DAO to FLASHINESS,

而 愚 之 始。

ér   *yú*   *zhī*   *shǐ.*
BUT   FOOLISHNESS   [PART]   BEGINNING.

BUT this is the BEGINNING OF FOOLISHNESS.

是 以 大 丈 夫 处 其 厚, 不 居

shì   *yǐ*   *dà*   *zhàng*   *fū*   *chǔ*   *qí*   *hòu,*   *bù*   *jū*
BE   WHY   GREAT   MAN   DEAL   ITS   PROFOUND,   NOT   DWELL

其 薄;

qí   *bó;*
ITS   THIN;

This IS WHY the GREAT MAN DEALS with the PROFOUND, but does NOT DWELL on the SUPERFICIAL;

处 其 实, 不 居 其 华。

chǔ   *qí*   *shí,*   *bù*   *jū*   *qí*   *huá.*
DEAL   ITS   SOLID,   NOT   DWELL   ITS   FLASHY.

HE DEALS with the SOLID, but does NOT DWELL on the FLASHY.

故 去 彼 取 此。

gù   *qù*   *bǐ*   *qǔ*   *cǐ.*
THEREFORE   GO   THAT   TAKE   THIS.

THEREFORE he LEAVES THAT and TAKES THIS.

昔　之　得　一　者：

xī　zhī　dé　yī　zhě:

PREVIOUSLY [PART] GAIN ONE [PART]:

These are the things WHICH have PREVIOUSLY GAINED the ONE:

天　得　一　以　清；

tiān　dé　yī　yǐ　qīng;

HEAVEN GAIN ONE [PART] CLEAR;

HEAVEN GAINED the ONE and BECAME CLEAR;

地　得　一　以　宁；

dì　dé　yī　yǐ　níng;

EARTH GAIN ONE [PART] PEACEFUL;

EARTH GAINED the ONE and BECAME PEACEFUL;

神　得　一　以　灵；

shén　dé　yī　yǐ　líng;

GOD GAIN ONE TAKE SPIRIT;

The GODS GAINED the ONE and ACQUIRED SPIRIT;

谷　得　一　以　盈；

gù　dé　yī　yǐ　yíng;

VALLEY GAIN ONE [PART] FULL;

The VALLEY GAINED the ONE and BECAME FULL;

万　物　得　一　以　生；

wàn　wù　dé　yī　yǐ　shēng;

TEN-THOUSAND THING GAIN ONE [PART] BIRTH;

ALL THINGS GAINED the ONE and WERE BORN;

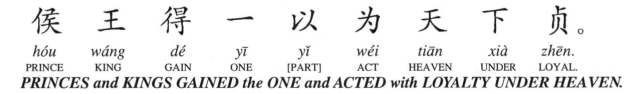

侯　王　得　一　以　为　天　下　贞。

hóu　wáng　dé　yī　yǐ　wéi　tiān　xià　zhēn.

PRINCE KING GAIN ONE [PART] ACT HEAVEN UNDER LOYAL.

PRINCES and KINGS GAINED the ONE and ACTED with LOYALTY UNDER HEAVEN.

其　　致　　之　　也　　谓：

qí　*zhì*　*zhī*　*yě*　*wèi:*
IT　RESULT　IT　[PART]　SAY:

In RESULT I SAY:

天　　无　　以　　清，　将　　恐　　裂；

tiān　*wú*　*yǐ*　*qīng,*　*jiāng*　*kǒng*　*liè;*
HEAVEN　NOT　TAKE　CLEAR,　WILL　FEAR　SPLIT;

If HEAVEN IS NOT CLEAR, I FEAR it WILL SPLIT;

地　　无　　以　　宁，　将　　恐　　废；

dì　*wú*　*yǐ*　*níng,*　*jiāng*　*kǒng*　*fèi;*
EARTH　NOT　TAKE　PEACEFUL,　WILL　FEAR　WASTE;

If the EARTH IS NOT PEACEFUL, I FEAR it WILL be WASTED;

神　　无　　以　　灵，　将　　恐　　歇；

shén　*wú*　*yǐ*　*líng,*　*jiāng*　*kǒng*　*xiē;*
GOD　NOT　TAKE　SPIRIT,　WILL　FEAR　REST;

If the GODS do NOT ACQUIRE SPIRIT, I FEAR they WILL be put to REST;

谷　　无　　以　　盈，　将　　恐　　竭；

gǔ　*wú*　*yǐ*　*yíng,*　*jiāng*　*kǒng*　*jié;*
VALLEY　NOT　TAKE　FULL,　WILL　FEAR　EXHAUST;

If the VALLEY IS NOT FULL, I FEAR it WILL be EXHAUSTED;

万　　物　　无　　以　　生，　将　　恐　　灭；

wàn　*wù*　*wú*　*yǐ*　*shēng,*　*jiāng*　*kǒng*　*miè;*
TEN-THOUSAND THING　NOT　TAKE　BIRTH,　WILL　FEAR　EXTINGUISH;

If ALL THINGS ARE NOT BORN, I FEAR they WILL be EXTINGUISHED;

侯	王	无	以	贞,	将	恐	蹶。
hóu	*wáng*	*wú*	*yǐ*	*zhēn,*	*jiāng*	*kǒng*	*jué.*
PRINCE	KING	NOT	[PART]	LOYAL,	WILL	FEAR	SETBACK.

If PRINCES and KINGS ARE NOT LOYAL, I FEAR there WILL be SETBACKS.

故	贵	以	贱	为	本;	高	以	下	为	基。
gù	*guì*	*yǐ*	*jiàn*	*wéi*	*běn;*	*gāo*	*yǐ*	*xià*	*wéi*	*jī.*
FOR	COSTLY	TAKE	HUMBLE	AS	ROOT;	HIGH	TAKE	LOW	AS	FOUNDATION.

FOR the COSTLY TAKES the HUMBLE AS its ROOT; the HIGH TAKES the LOW AS its FOUNDATION.

是	以	侯	王	自	称	孤、	寡、	不	谷。
shì	*yǐ*	*hóu*	*wáng*	*zì*	*chēng*	*gū,*	*guǎ,*	*bù*	*gǔ.*
BE	WHY	PRINCE	KING	SELF	CALL	SOLITARY,	SCANT,	NOT	VALLEY.

This IS WHY PRINCES and KINGS CALL THEMSELVES "SOLITARY," "SCANT," and "NOT ABUNDANT."

此	非	以	贱	为	本	邪?	非	乎?
cǐ	*fēi*	*yǐ*	*jiàn*	*wéi*	*běn*	*yé?*	*fēi*	*hū?*
THIS	NOT	TAKE	HUMBLE	AS	ROOT	[PART]?	NOT	[PART]?

Does the COSTLY NOT TAKE the HUMBLE AS its ROOT? Does it NOT?

故	至	誉	无	誉。
gù	*zhì*	*yù*	*wú*	*yù.*
THEREFORE	EXTREME	PRAISE	NOT	PRAISE.

THEREFORE EXTREME PRAISE is NOT PRAISE.

是	故	不	欲	琭	琭	如	玉,	珞	珞
shì	*gù*	*bù*	*yù*	*lù*	*lù*	*rú*	*yù,*	*luò*	*luò*
BE	REASON	NOT	DESIRE	EXQUISITE		LIKE	JADE,	ORNATE	

如	石。
rú	*shí.*
LIKE	STONE.

This IS the REASON one should NOT DESIRE to be EXQUISITE LIKE JADE or ORNATE like jewelry of STONE.

反　者　道　之　动;

fǎn　zhě　dào　zhī　dòng;
RETURN　[PART]　DAO　[PART]　MOTION;

RETURNING is the MOTION OF the DAO;

弱　者　道　之　用。

ruò　zhě　dào　zhī　yòng.
WEAK　[PART]　DAO　[PART]　USE.

WEAKNESS is the USE OF the DAO.

天　下　万　物　生　于　有;

tiān　xià　wàn　wù　shēng　yú　yǒu;
HEAVEN　UNDER　TEN-THOUSAND　THING　BORN　FROM　EXISTENCE;

ALL THINGS UNDER HEAVEN are BORN OF EXISTENCE;

有　生　于　无。

yǒu　shēng　yú　wú.
EXISTENCE　BORN　FROM　NOTHINGNESS.

EXISTENCE is BORN OF NOTHINGNESS.

Chapter 41

上　士　闻　道，勤　而　行　之；

shàng　shì　wén　dào，qín　ér　xíng　zhī；

SUPERIOR　SCHOLAR　HEAR　DAO，DILIGENTLY　AND　EXECUTE　IT；

When the SUPERIOR SCHOLAR HEARS the DAO, he DILIGENTLY EXECUTES IT;

中　士　闻　道，若　存　若　亡；

zhōng　shì　wén　dào，ruò　cún　ruò　wáng；

AVERAGE　SCHOLAR　HEAR　DAO，SEEM　PRESERVE　SEEM　LOSE；

When the AVERAGE SCHOLAR HEARS the DAO, it is SOMETIMES PRESERVED and SOMETIMES LOST;

下　士　闻　道，大　而　笑　之。

xià　shì　wén　dào，dà　ér　xiào　zhī.

INFERIOR　SCHOLAR　HEAR　DAO，GREATLY　[PART]　LAUGH　IT.

When the INFERIOR SCHOLAR HEARS the DAO, he LAUGHS at IT GREATLY.

不　笑　不　足　以　为　道。

bú　xiào　bù　zú　yǐ　wéi　dào.

NOT　LAUGH　NOT　ENOUGH　TO　ACT　DAO.

If one does NOT LAUGH, one will be UNABLE TO ENACT the DAO.

故　建　言　有　之：

gù　jiàn　yán　yǒu　zhī：

THEREFORE　ESTABLISH　SPEECH　EXIST　IT：

THEREFORE these ESTABLISHED SAYINGS EXIST:

明　道　若　昧；进　道　若　退；

míng　dào　ruò　mèi；jìn　dào　ruò　tuì；

BRIGHT　DAO　SEEM　DARK；ADVANCE　DAO　SEEM　RETREAT；

The BRIGHT DAO SEEMS DARK; the ADVANCING DAO SEEMS to RETREAT;

夷　道　若　颣；　上　德　若　谷；

yí　dào　ruò　lèi;　shàng　dé　ruò　gǔ;

SMOOTH　DAO　SEEM　FLAWED;　SUPERIOR　VIRTUE　SEEM　VALLEY;

The SMOOTH DAO SEEMS FLAWED; SUPERIOR VIRTUE SEEMS like a VALLEY;

大　白　若　辱；　广　德　若　不　足；

dà　bái　ruò　rǔ;　guǎng　dé　ruò　bù　zú;

GREAT　WHITE　SEEM　BLACK;　WIDE　VIRTUE　SEEM　NOT　SUFFICIENT;

PERFECT WHITENESS SEEMS like BLACKNESS; EXTENSIVE VIRTUE SEEMS INSUFFICIENT;

建　德　若　偷；　质　真　若　渝。

jiàn　dé　ruò　tōu;　zhì　zhēn　ruò　yú.

VIGOROUS　VIRTUE　SEEM　LISTLESS;　SIMPLE　TRUTH　SEEM　CHANGE.

VIGOROUS VIRTUE SEEMS LISTLESS; the SIMPLE TRUTH SEEMS CHANGEABLE.

大　方　无　隅；　大　器　晚　成；

dà　fāng　wú　yú;　dà　qì　wǎn　chéng;

GREAT　SQUARE　NOT　CORNER;　GREAT　IMPLEMENT　LATE　ACHIEVE;

The PERFECT SQUARE has NO CORNERS; the PERFECT IMPLEMENT is COMPLETED LAST;

大　音　希　声；　大　象　无　形。

dà　yīn　xī　shēng;　dà　xiàng　wú　xíng.

GREAT　NOTE　THIN　SOUND;　GREAT　IMAGE　NOT　FORM.

The PERFECT NOTE has a THIN SOUND; the PERFECT IMAGE has NO FORM.

道　隐　无　名。

dào　yǐn　wú　míng.

DAO　HIDDEN　NOT　NAME.

The DAO is HIDDEN and UNNAMED.

夫　唯　道，　善　贷　且　成。

fú　wéi　dào,　shàn　dài　qiě　chéng.

FOR　DAO,　ADEPT　NOURISH　AND　ACHIEVE.

FOR the DAO is ADEPT at NOURISHING all things AND brings them to FRUITION.

Chapter 42

道　生　一；　一　生　二；

dào　shēng　yī;　yī　shēng　èr;
DAO　BEAR　ONE;　ONE　BEAR　TWO;

The DAO gives BIRTH to ONE; ONE gives BIRTH to TWO;

二　生　三；　三　生　万　物。

èr　shēng　sān;　sān　shēng　wàn　wù.
TWO　BEAR　THREE;　THREE　BEAR　TEN-THOUSAND　THING.

TWO gives BIRTH to THREE; THREE gives BIRTH to ALL THINGS.

万　物　负　阴　而　抱　阳；

wàn　wù　fù　yīn　ér　bào　yáng;
TEN-THOUSAND　THING　CARRY　YIN　AND　EMBRACE　YANG;

ALL THINGS CARRY YIN AND EMBRACE YANG;

冲　气　以　为　和。

chōng　qì　yǐ　wéi　hé.
MIX　FORCE　TO　SERVE-AS　HARMONY.

All things MIX these FORCES TO CREATE HARMONY.

人　之　所　恶：唯　孤、寡、不　谷。

rén　zhī　suǒ　wù:　wéi　gū,　guǎ,　bù　gǔ.
PEOPLE　[PART]　WHAT　LOATHE:　ONLY　SOLITARY,　SCANT,　NOT　VALLEY.

This is WHAT the PEOPLE LOATHE: ONLY "SOLITARY," "SCANT," and "NOT ABUNDANT."

而　王　公　以　为　称。

ér　wáng-　gōng　yǐ　wéi　chēng.
YET　KING-　DUKE　TAKE　AS　CALL.

YET the NOBLES TAKE these terms AS their TITLES.

故　物　或　损　之　而　益，

gù　wù　huò　sǔn　zhī　ér　yì,
SO　THING　EITHER　REDUCE　THEM　BUT　INCREASE,

SO as for THINGS: one may REDUCE THEM, BUT they will INCREASE,

或　益　之　而　损。

huò　yì　zhī　ér　sǔn.
OR　INCREASE　THEM　BUT　REDUCE.

OR one may INCREASE THEM, BUT they will be REDUCED.

人　之　所　教，我　亦　教　之。

rén　zhī　suǒ　jiào,　wǒ　yì　jiào　zhī.
PERSON　[PART]　WHAT　TEACH,　I　ALSO　TEACH　IT.

WHAT OTHERS TEACH, I ALSO TEACH.

强　梁　者　不　得　其　死：

qiáng　liáng　zhě,　bù　dé　qí　sǐ:
FORCE　BEAM　[PART],　NOT　GAIN　THEIR　DEATH:

Those WHO FORCE the BEAM do NOT GAIN a good DEATH:

吾　将　以　为　教　父。

wú　jiāng　yǐ　wéi　jiào　fù.
I　WILL　TAKE　AS　TEACH　FATHER.

I WILL TAKE this AS the BASIS of my TEACHING.

Chapter 43

天　下　之　至　柔，

tiān *xià* *zhī* *zhì* *róu,*
HEAVEN　UNDER　[PART]　MOST　SOFT,

The SOFTEST things UNDER HEAVEN

驰　骋　天　下　之　至　坚。

chí *chěng* *tiān* *xià* *zhī* *zhì* *jiān.*
GALLOP　HEAVEN　UNDER　[PART]　MOST　HARD.

PERMEATE the HARDEST things UNDER HEAVEN.

无　有　入　无　间。

wú *yǒu* *rù* *wú* *jiàn.*
NOT　HAVE　ENTER　NOT　SPACE.

That which HAS NO form can ENTER where there is NO SPACE.

吾　是　以　知　无　为　之　有　益。

wú *shì* *yǐ* *zhī* *wú* *wéi* *zhī* *yǒu* *yì.*
I　BE　WHY　KNOW　NOT　ACT　[PART]　HAVE　BENEFIT.

This IS WHY I KNOW that NON-ACTION IS BENEFICIAL.

不　言　之　教，无　为　之　益:

bù *yán* *zhī* *jiào,* *wú* *wéi* *zhī* *yì:*
NOT　SPEAK　[PART]　TEACH,　NOT　ACT　[PART]　BENEFIT:

TEACHING by NOT SPEAKING and the BENEFIT OF NON-ACTION:

天　下　希　及　之。

tiān *xià* *xī* *jí* *zhī.*
HEAVEN　UNDER　FEW　ATTAIN　THEM.

UNDER HEAVEN FEW ATTAIN THEM.

名　与　身:　孰　亲?

míng	yǔ	shēn:	shú	qīn?
FAME	OR	LIFE:	WHICH	INTIMATE?

FAME OR LIFE: WHICH is more INTIMATELY desired?

身　与　货:　孰　多?

shēn	yǔ	huò:	shú	duō?
LIFE	OR	COMMODITY:	WHICH	MORE?

LIFE OR COMMODITIES: WHICH is GREATER?

得　与　亡:　孰　病?

dé	yǔ	wáng:	shú	bìng?
GAIN	OR	LOSE:	WHICH	HARMFUL?

GAIN OR LOSS: WHICH is more HARMFUL?

甚　爱　必　大　费;　多　藏　必　厚　亡。

shèn	ài	bì	dà	fèi;	duō	cáng	bì	hòu	wáng.
EXTREMELY	LOVE	MUST	GREATLY	PAY;	MUCH	HOARD	MUST	PROFOUNDLY	LOSE.

Those who LOVE EXTREMELY MUST PAY DEARLY; those who HOARD MANY things MUST LOSE PROFOUNDLY.

故　知　足　不　辱;

gù	zhī	zú	bù	rǔ;
THEREFORE	KNOW	ENOUGH	NOT	DISGRACE;

THEREFORE those who KNOW when they have ENOUGH will NOT be DISGRACED;

知　止　不　殆;　可　以　长　久。

zhī	zhǐ	bú	dài;	kě	yǐ	cháng	jiǔ.
KNOW	STOP	NOT	HARM;	CAN		LONG	LONG-TIME.

Those who KNOW when to STOP will NOT be HARMED; they CAN LONG CONTINUE.

Chapter 45

大　成　若　缺，　其　用　不　弊。
dà　*chéng*　*ruò*　*quē,*　*qí*　*yòng*　*bú*　*bì.*
GREAT　ACHIEVE　SEEM　DEFICIENT,　IT　USE　NOT　HARM.

GREAT ACHIEVEMENT SEEMS DEFICIENT, but if one USES IT, it will NOT be HARMED.

大　盈　若　冲，　其　用　不　穷。
dà　*yíng*　*ruò*　*chōng,*　*qí*　*yòng*　*bù*　*qióng.*
GREAT　FULL　SEEM　EMPTY,　IT　USE　NOT　EXHAUSTED.

GREAT FULLNESS SEEMS EMPTY, but if one USES IT, it will NOT be EXHAUSTED.

大　直　若　屈；　大　巧　若　拙；
dà　*zhí*　*ruò*　*qū;*　*dà*　*qiǎo*　*ruò*　*zhuō;*
GREAT　STRAIGHT　SEEM　CROOKED;　GREAT　SKILL　SEEM　AWKWARD;

GREAT STRAIGHTNESS SEEMS CROOKED; GREAT SKILL SEEMS AWKWARD;

大　辩　若　讷。
dà　*biàn*　*ruò*　*nè.*
GREAT　ARGUMENTATION　SEEM　INARTICULATE.

GREAT ARGUMENTATION SEEMS INARTICULATE.

躁　胜　寒；　静　胜　热。
zào　*shèng*　*hán;*　*jìng*　*shèng*　*rè.*
IMPETUOUS　CONQUER　COLD;　CALM　CONQUERS　HEAT.

IMPETUOUS motion CONQUERS COLD; CALM CONQUERS HEAT.

清　静　为　天　下　正。
qīng-　*jìng*　*wéi*　*tiān*　*xià*　*zhèng.*
CLEAR-　CALM　ACT　HEAVEN　UNDER　RIGHT.

TRANQUILITY ACTS to set RIGHT all things UNDER HEAVEN.

Chapter 46

天　下　有　道，却　走　马　以　粪；

tiān *xià* *yǒu* *dào,* *què* *zǒu-* *mǎ* *yǐ* *fèn;*
HEAVEN　UNDER　EXIST　DAO,　AND　WALK-　HORSE　TAKE　MANURE;

When the DAO REIGNS UNDER HEAVEN, WORKHORSES MANURE the fields;

天　下　无　道，戎　马　生　于　郊。

tiān *xià* *wú* *dào,* *róng* *mǎ* *shēng* *yú* *jiāo.*
HEAVEN　UNDER　NOT　DAO,　ARMY　HORSE　BEAR　IN　OUTSKIRTS.

When the DAO does NOT reign UNDER HEAVEN, ARMY HORSES are BRED IN the OUTSKIRTS.

祸　莫　大　于　不　知　足；

huò *mò* *dà* *yú* *bù* *zhī* *zú;*
DISASTER　NOT　GREATER　THAN　NOT　KNOW　ENOUGH;

There is NO GREATER DISASTER THAN NOT KNOWING when one has ENOUGH;

咎　莫　大　于　欲　得。

jiù *mò* *dà* *yú* *yù* *dé.*
FAULT　NOT　GREATER　THAN　DESIRE　GAIN.

There is NO GREATER FAULT THAN the DESIRE for GAIN.

故　知　足　之　足，常　足　矣。

gù *zhī* *zú* *zhī* *zú,* *cháng* *zú* *yǐ.*
THEREFORE　KNOW　SUFFICIENT　[PART]　SUFFICIENT,　ALWAYS　ENOUGH　[PART].

THEREFORE those who KNOW the SUFFICIENCY OF SUFFICIENCY ALWAYS have ENOUGH.

Chapter 47

不　出　户，知　天　下；
bù　chū　hù,　zhī　tiān　xià;
NOT　EXIT　DOOR,　KNOW　HEAVEN　UNDER;

WITHOUT EXITING through the DOOR, one can KNOW all things UNDER HEAVEN;

不　窥　牖，见　天　道。
bù　kuī　yǒu,　jiàn　tiān　dào.
NOT　PEER　WINDOW,　SEE　HEAVEN　DAO.

WITHOUT PEERING through the WINDOW, one can SEE the DAO of HEAVEN.

其　出　弥　远，其　知　弥　少。
qí　chū　mí　yuán,　qí　zhī　mí　shǎo.
ONE　EXIT　MORE　FAR,　ONE　KNOW　MORE　FEW.

The FURTHER ONE GOES, the LESS ONE KNOWS.

是　以　圣　人　不　行　而　知；
shì　yǐ　shèng-　rén　bù　xíng　ér　zhī;
BE　WHY　SAGACIOUS-　PERSON　NOT　TRAVEL　BUT　KNOW;

This IS WHY the SAGE does NOT TRAVEL, BUT he KNOWS;

不　见　而　明；不　为　而　成。
bú　jiàn　ér　míng;　bù　wéi　ér　chéng.
NOT　SEE　BUT　UNDERSTAND;　NOT　ACT　BUT　ACHIEVE.

He does NOT SEE, BUT he UNDERSTANDS; he does NOT ACT, BUT he ACHIEVES.

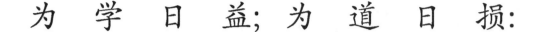

为　学　日　益；为　道　日　损：

wéi　xué　rì　yì;　wéi　dào　rì　sǔn:

ACT　SCHOLARSHIP　DAY　INCREASE;　ACT　DAO　DAY　REDUCE:

In UNDERTAKING SCHOLARSHIP there are DAILY INCREASES; in ENACTING the DAO there are DAILY REDUCTIONS:

损　之　又　损，以　至　于　无　为。

sǔn　zhī　yòu　sǔn,　yǐ　zhì　yú　wú　wéi.

REDUCE　IT　AGAIN　REDUCE,　[PART]　UNTIL　AT　NOT　ACT.

REDUCTIONS and MORE REDUCTIONS, UNTIL one arrives AT NON-ACTION.

无　为　而　无　不　为。

wú　wéi　ér　wú　bù　wéi.

NOT　ACT　BUT　NOT　NOT　ACT.

The dao does NOT ACT, BUT there is NOTHING that it does NOT ACHIEVE.

取　天　下　常　以　无　事；

qǔ　tiān　xià　cháng　yǐ　wú　shì;

TAKE　HEAVEN　UNDER　ALWAYS　TAKE　NOT　AFFAIR;

In RULING all things UNDER HEAVEN one should ALWAYS APPLY NON-INTERFERENCE;

及　其　有　事，不　足　以　取　天　下。

jí　qí　yǒu　shì,　bù　zú　yǐ　qǔ　tiān　xià.

REACH　THEM　HAVE　AFFAIR,　NOT　ENOUGH　TO　TAKE　HEAVEN　UNDER.

If one APPROACHES THINGS INTERFERINGLY, one will be UNABLE TO RULE all things UNDER HEAVEN.

Chapter 49

圣 人 常 无 心;

shèng- rén cháng wú xīn;
SAGACIOUS- PERSON ALWAYS NOT HEART;

The SAGE NEVER follows his own HEART;

以 百 姓 之 心 为 心。

yǐ bǎi xìng zhī xīn wéi xīn.
TAKE HUNDRED SURNAME [PART] HEART AS HEART.

He TAKES the PEOPLE'S HEART AS his own HEART.

善 者, 吾 善 之;

shàn zhě, wú shàn zhī;
KIND [PART], I KIND THEM;

As for the KIND, I am KIND to THEM;

不 善 者, 吾 亦 善 之: 德 善。

bú shàn zhě, wú yì shàn zhī: dé shàn.
NOT KIND [PART], I ALSO KIND THEM: VIRTUE KIND.

As for the UNKIND, I am ALSO KIND to THEM: VIRTUE is KIND.

信 者, 吾 信 之;

xìn zhě, wú xìn zhī;
TRUST [PART], I TRUST THEM;

As for the TRUSTING, I TRUST THEM;

不 信 者, 吾 亦 信 之: 德 信。

bú xìn zhě, wú yì xìn zhī: dé xìn.
NOT TRUST [PART], I ALSO TRUST THEM: VIRTUE TRUST.

As for those WHO are NOT TRUSTING, I ALSO TRUST THEM: VIRTUE is TRUSTING.

圣　　人　　在　　天　　下，　歙　　歙　　焉。

shèng- *rén* *zài* *tiān* *xià,* *xī* *xī* *yān.*
SAGACIOUS- PERSON IN HEAVEN UNDER, INHALE [PART].

When the SAGE APPEARS UNDER HEAVEN, he DRAWS BACK.

为　　天　　下　　浑　　其　　心。

wéi *tiān* *xià* *hún* *qí* *xīn.*
ACT HEAVEN UNDER SIMPLE HIS HEART.

When he ACTS UNDER HEAVEN he makes HIS HEART SIMPLE.

百　　姓　　皆　　注　　其　　耳　　目；

bǎi *xìng* *jiē* *zhù* *qí* *ěr* *mù;*
HUNDRED SURNAME ALL CONCENTRATE THEIR EAR EYE;

The PEOPLE ALL CONCENTRATE THEIR EARS and EYES on him;

圣　　人　　皆　　孩　　之。

shèng- *rén* *jiē* *hái* *zhī.*
SAGACIOUS- PERSON ALL CHILD THEM.

Toward ALL of THEM, the SAGE acts like a CHILD.

Chapter 50

出　生　入　死，
chū　shēng　rù　sǐ,
EXIT　BORN　ENTER　DIE,
In being BORN and in DYING,

生　之　徒，十　有　三；
shēng　zhī　tú,　shí　yǒu　sān;
LIFE　[PART]　FOLLOWER,　TEN　EXIST　THREE;
As for the FOLLOWERS OF LIFE, in TEN there ARE THREE;

死　之　徒，十　有　三；
sǐ　zhī　tú,　shí　yǒu　sān;
DEATH　[PART]　FOLLOWER,　TEN　EXIST　THREE;
As for the FOLLOWERS OF DEATH, in TEN there ARE THREE;

人　之　生，动　之　于　死　地，
rén　zhī　shēng,　dòng　zhī　yú　sǐ　dì,
PERSON　[PART]　LIFE,　MOVE　IT　TO　DEATH　REALM,
As for those who take THEIR LIFE and RELINQUISH IT TO the REALM of DEATH,

亦　十　有　三。
yì　shí　yǒu　sān.
ALSO　TEN　EXIST　THREE.
In TEN there ARE ALSO THREE.

夫　何　故？以　其　生，生　之　厚。
fú　hé　gù?　yǐ　qí　shēng,　shēng　zhī　hòu.
SO　WHAT　REASON?　USE　THEIR　LIFE,　LIFE　[PART]　THICK.
WHAT is the REASON? They USE THEIR LIFE to pursue LIFE'S GROSSNESS.

盖　闻　善　摄　生　者，

gài　wén　shàn　shè　shēng　zhě,

SO　HEAR　GOOD　ARRANGE　LIFE　[PART],

BUT those WHO ATTEND to GOODNESS in ARRANGING their LIFE

陆　生　不　遇　兕　虎。

lù　shēng　bú　yù　sì　hǔ.

ROAD　WALK　NOT　ENCOUNTER　RHINOCEROS　TIGER.

ENCOUNTER NO RHINOCEROS or TIGER when they WALK on the ROAD.

入　军　不　被　甲　兵。

rù　jūn　bú　bèi　jiǎ　bīng.

ENTER　ARMY　NOT　BY　ARMOR　WEAPON.

When they ENTER the ARMY, they are NOT harmed BY MILITARY WEAPONS.

兕　无　所　投　其　角。

sì　wú　suǒ　tóu　qí　jiǎo.

RHINOCEROS　NOT　WHERE　THRUST　ITS　HORN.

The RHINOCEROS has NOWHERE to THRUST ITS HORN

虎　无　所　措　其　爪。

hǔ　wú　suǒ　cuò　qí　zhǎo.

TIGER　NOT　WHERE　PLACE　ITS　CLAW.

The TIGER has NOWHERE to PLACE ITS CLAWS.

兵　无　所　容　其　刃。

bīng　wú　suǒ　róng　qí　rèn.

WEAPON　NOT　WHERE　HOLD　ITS　BLADE.

A WEAPON has NOWHERE to INSERT ITS BLADE.

夫　何　故？以　其　无　死　地。

fú　hé　gù?　yǐ　qí　wú　sǐ　dì.

SO　WHAT　REASON?　BECAUSE　THEY　NOT　DEATH　PLACE.

WHAT is the REASON? BECAUSE THEY have NO PLACE for DEATH.

Chapter 51

道　生　之;　德　畜　之;

dào　shēng　zhī;　dé　xù　zhī;
DAO　BEAR　THEM;　VIRTUE　REAR　THEM;

The DAO gives BIRTH to the all THINGS; VIRTUE REARS THEM;

物　形　之;　势　成　之。

wù　xíng　zhī;　shì　chéng　zhī.
SUBSTANCE　FORM　THEM;　CIRCUMSTANCE　COMPLETE　THEM.

SUBSTANCE FORMS THEM; CIRCUMSTANCES COMPLETE THEM.

是　以　万　物　莫　不　尊　道　而　贵

shì　yǐ　wàn　wù　mò　bù　zūn　dào　ér　guì
BE　WHY　TEN-THOUSAND　THING　NOT　NOT　HONOR　DAO　AND　ESTEEM

德。

dé.
VIRTUE.

This IS WHY among the TEN THOUSAND THINGS there is NOT one that does NOT HONOR the DAO AND ESTEEM VIRTUE.

道　之　尊,　德　之　贵,

dào　zhī　zūn,　dé　zhī　guì,
DAO　[PART]　HONOR,　VIRTUE　[PART]　ESTEEM,

They HONOR the DAO and ESTEEM VIRTUE,

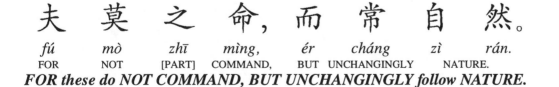

夫　莫　之　命,　而　常　自　然。

fú　mò　zhī　mìng,　ér　cháng　zì　rán.
FOR　NOT　[PART]　COMMAND,　BUT　UNCHANGINGLY　NATURE.

FOR these do NOT COMMAND, BUT UNCHANGINGLY follow NATURE.

故　道　生　之；　德　畜　之，
gù　dào　shēng　zhī;　dé　xù　zhī,
THEREFORE　DAO　BEAR　THEM;　VIRTUE　REAR　THEM,

THEREFORE the DAO gives BIRTH to all THINGS; VIRTUE REARS THEM,

长　之　育　之；　亭　之　毒　之；
zhǎng　zhī　yù　zhī;　tíng　zhī　dú　zhī;
FURTHER　THEM　GROW　THEM;　RAISE　THEM　RIPEN　THEM;

FURTHERS THEM and lets THEM GROW; RAISES THEM and lets THEM RIPEN;

养　之　覆　之。
yǎng　zhī　fù　zhī.
FOSTER　THEM　PROTECT　THEM.

FOSTERS THEM and PROTECTS THEM.

生　而　不　有；　为　而　不　恃；
shēng　ér　bù　yǒu;　wéi　ér　bú　shì;
BEAR　BUT　NOT　POSSESS;　ACT　BUT　NOT　DEPEND;

To give BIRTH BUT NOT POSSESS; to ACT BUT NOT DEPEND;

长　而　不　宰：　是　谓　玄　德。
zhǎng　ér　bù　zǎi:　shì　wèi　xuán　dé.
FURTHER　BUT　NOT　RULE:　BE　CALL　PROFOUND　VIRTUE.

To FURTHER BUT NOT RULE: this IS CALLED "PROFOUND VIRTUE."

Chapter 52

天　　下　　有　　始；　以　　为　　天　　下　　母。
tiān　　*xià*　　*yǒu*　　*shǐ;*　　*yǐ*　　*wéi*　　*tiān*　　*xià*　　*mǔ*
HEAVEN　UNDER　HAVE　BEGINNING;　[PART]　ACT　HEAVEN　UNDER　MOTHER.

All things UNDER HEAVEN HAVE a BEGINNING; it ACTS as the MOTHER of all things UNDER HEAVEN.

既　　得　　其　　母，　以　　知　　其　　子；
jì　　*dé*　　*qí*　　*mǔ,*　　*yǐ*　　*zhī*　　*qí*　　*zǐ;*
SINCE　GAIN　THEIR　MOTHER,　[PART]　KNOW　HER　OFFSPRING;

IF one GAINS the MOTHER one CAN KNOW HER OFFSPRING;

既　　知　　其　　子，　复　　守　　其　　母。
jì　　*zhī*　　*qí*　　*zǐ,*　　*fù*　　*shǒu*　　*qí*　　*mǔ.*
SINCE　KNOW　HER　OFFSPRING,　AGAIN　PRESERVE　THEIR　MOTHER.

IF one KNOWS HER OFFSPRING, one can AGAIN PRESERVE the MOTHER.

没　　身　　不　　殆。
mò　　*shēn*　　*bú*　　*dài.*
END　LIFE　NOT　HARM.

Unto the END of LIFE there will be NO HARM.

塞　　其　　兑，　闭　　其　　门，
sāi　　*qí*　　*duì,*　　*bì*　　*qí*　　*mén,*
STOP-UP　ONE'S　EXCHANGE,　CLOSE　ONE'S　DOOR,

If one STOPS INTERACTING and CLOSES ONE'S DOOR,

终　　身　　不　　勤。
zhōng　　*shēn*　　*bù*　　*qín.*
END　LIFE　NOT　PERSISTENT.

Unto the END of LIFE there will be NO PERSISTENT troubles.

开　其　兑，济　起　身，终　身　不　救。
kāi　qí　duì,　jì　qí　shēn,　zhōng　shēn　bú　jiù.
OPEN　ONE'S　EXCHANGE,　BENEFIT　ONE'S　LIFE,　END　LIFE　NOT　SAVE.

If one KEEPS INTERACTING and busies ONE'S LIFE seeking BENEFITS, unto the END of LIFE there will be NO SALVATION.

见　小　日　明；守　柔　日　强。
jiàn　xiǎo　yuē　míng;　shǒu　róu　yuē　qiáng.
SEE　SMALL　CALL　BRIGHT;　PRESERVE　SOFT　CALL　STRONG.

SEEING the SMALL is CALLED "BRIGHTNESS;" PRESERVING the SOFT is CALLED "STRENGTH."

用　其　光，复　归　其　明，
yòng　qí　guāng,　fù　guī　qí　míng,
USE　ITS　LIGHT,　AGAIN　RETURN　ITS　BRIGHT,

If one USES the LIGHT, one can AGAIN RETURN to BRIGHTNESS,

无　遗　身　殃：是　为　袭　常。
wú　yí　shēn　yāng:　shì　wéi　xí　cháng.
NOT　HAND-DOWN　BODY　DISASTER:　BE　AS　PERPETUATE　UNCHANGING.

NOT HANDING DOWN to oneself one's OWN DEMISE: this IS to PERPETUATE the UNCHANGING.

Chapter 53

使　我　介　然　有　知，

shǐ　*wǒ*　*jiè*　*rán*　*yǒu*　*zhī,*
CAUSE　I　ANY　POSSESS　KNOWLEDGE,

IF I POSSESS ANY KNOWLEDGE at all,

行　于　大　道；唯　施　是　畏。

xíng　*yú*　*dà*　*dào;*　*wéi*　*shī*　*shì*　*wèi.*
WALK　ON　GREAT　ROAD;　ONLY　STRAY　BE　FEAR.

I will WALK ON the GREAT ROAD of the dao; my ONLY FEAR will BE STRAYING from it.

大　道　甚　夷，而　人　好　径。

dà　*dào*　*shèn*　*yí,*　*ér*　*rén*　*hào*　*jìng.*
GREAT　ROAD　VERY　SAFE,　BUT　PEOPLE　PREFER　PATH.

The GREAT ROAD of the dao is VERY SAFE, BUT PEOPLE PREFER the narrow PATH.

朝　甚　除：田　甚　芜，

cháo　*shèn*　*chú:*　*tián*　*shèn*　*wú,*
COURT　VERY　ELIMINATE:　FIELD　VERY　OVERGROWN,

The royal COURT is VERY WASTEFUL: the FIELDS are VERY OVERGROWN,

仓　甚　虚，服　文　采；

cāng　*shèn*　*xū,*　*fú*　*wén*　*cǎi;*
STOREHOUSE　VERY　EMPTY,　CLOTHING　RICH　BRIGHT;

The STOREHOUSES are BARREN, yet the courtiers' CLOTHING is RICHLY and BRIGHTLY colored;

带　利　剑，厌　饮　食。

dài　*lì*　*jiàn,*　*yàn*　*yǐn*　*shí.*
WEAR　SHARP　SWORD,　SATED　DRINK　EAT.

They WEAR SHARP SWORDS, and are SATED from DRINKING and EATING.

財　　貨　　有　　馀，

cái   *huò*   *yǒu*   *yú.*

WEALTH   GOODS   POSSESS   EXCESS.

They POSSESS WEALTH and GOODS in EXCESS.

是　　謂　　盗　　竽。

shì   *wèi*   *dào*   *yú.*

BE   CALL   BANDIT   REED.

Such people ARE CALLED "BANDITS whose bragging is like the playing of REEDS."

非　　道　　也　　哉！

fēi   *dào*   *yě*   *zāi!*

NOT   DAO   [PART]   [PART]!

This is NOT the DAO!

Chapter 54

善　建　者，　不　拔；

shàn　*jiàn*　*zhě,*　*bù*　*bá;*

WELL　CONSTRUCT　[PART],　NOT　LIFT;

WHAT is WELL-CONSTRUCTED CANNOT be LIFTED away;

善　抱　者，　不　脱：

shàn　*bào*　*zhě,*　*bù*　*tuō:*

WELL　EMBRACE　[PART],　NOT　REMOVE:

WHAT is WELL-EMBRACED CANNOT be REMOVED:

子　孙　以　祭　祀　不　辍。

zǐ　*sūn*　*yǐ*　*jì*　*sì*　*bú*　*chuò.*

SON　GRANDSON　UNDERTAKE　SACRIFICE　NOT　CEASE.

SONS and GRANDSONS will UNDERTAKE SACRIFICIAL rites UNCEASINGLY.

修　之　于　身，　其　德　乃　真；

xiū　*zhī*　*yú*　*shēn,*　*qí*　*dé*　*nǎi*　*zhēn;*

CULTIVATE　IT　IN　BODY,　ONE'S　VIRTUE　BE　TRUE;

CULTIVATE THIS IN the INDIVIDUAL, and the INDIVIDUAL'S VIRTUE will BE TRUE;

修　之　于　家，　其　德　乃　馀；

xiū　*zhī*　*yú*　*jiā,*　*qí*　*dé*　*nǎi*　*yú;*

CULTIVATE　IT　IN　FAMILY,　ITS　VIRTUE　BE　EXTRA;

CULTIVATE IT IN the FAMILY, and the FAMILY'S VIRTUE will BE PLENTIFUL;

修　之　于　乡，　其　德　乃　长；

xiū　*zhī*　*yú*　*xiāng,*　*qí*　*dé*　*nǎi*　*cháng;*

CULTIVATE　IT　IN　VILLAGE,　ITS　VIRTUE　BE　LASTING;

CULTIVATE IT IN the VILLAGE, and the VILLAGE'S VIRTUE will BE LASTING;

修 之 于 邦, 其 德 乃 丰;

xiū *zhī* *yú* *bāng,* *qí* *dé* *nǎi* *fēng;*

CULTIVATE IT IN NATION, ITS VIRTUE BE ABUNDANT;

CULTIVATE IT IN the NATION, and the NATION'S VIRTUE will BE ABUNDANT;

修 之 于 天 下, 其 德 乃 普。

xiū *zhī* *yú* *tiān* *xià,* *qí* *dé* *nǎi* *pǔ.*

CULTIVATE IT IN HEAVEN UNDER, THEIR VIRTUE BE UNIVERSAL.

CULTIVATE IT IN all things UNDER HEAVEN, and THEIR VIRTUE will BE UNIVERSAL.

故 以 身 观 身; 以 家 观 家;

gù *yǐ* *shēn* *guān* *shēn;* *yǐ* *jiā* *guān* *jiā;*

THEREFORE TAKE BODY OBSERVE BODY; TAKE FAMILY OBSERVE FAMILY;

THEREFORE TAKE the viewpoint of the INDIVIDUAL to OBSERVE the INDIVIDUAL; TAKE the viewpoint of the FAMILY to OBSERVE the FAMILY;

以 乡 观 乡; 以 邦 观 邦;

yǐ *xiāng* *guān* *xiāng;* *yǐ* *bāng* *guān* *bāng;*

TAKE VILLAGE OBSERVE VILLAGE; TAKE NATION OBSERVE NATION;

TAKE the viewpoint of the VILLAGE to OBSERVE the VILLAGE; TAKE the viewpoint of the NATION to OBSERVE the NATION;

以 天 下 观 天 下。

yǐ *tiān* *xià* *guān* *tiān* *xià.*

TAKE HEAVEN UNDER OBSERVE HEAVEN UNDER.

TAKE the viewpoint of all things UNDER HEAVEN to OBSERVE all things UNDER HEAVEN.

吾 何 以 知 天 下 然 哉? 以 此。

wú *hé* *yǐ* *zhī* *tiān* *xià* *rán* *zāi?* *yǐ* *cǐ.*

I HOW [PART] KNOW HEAVEN UNDER NATURE [PART]? USE THIS.

HOW do I KNOW the NATURE of all things UNDER HEAVEN? I USE THIS method.

Chapter 55

含　德　之　厚，比　于　赤　子。

hán　dé　zhī　hòu,　bǐ　yú　chì　zǐ.
HOLD　VIRTUE　[PART]　PROFOUND,　COMPARE　TO　BARE-RED　SON.

Those who HOLD within them the PROFUNDITY OF VIRTUE can be COMPARED TO a BABY BOY.

毒　虫　不　螫；猛　兽　不　据；

dú　chóng　bú　shì;　méng　shòu　bú　jù;
POISONOUS　INSECT　NOT　STING;　SAVAGE　BEAST　NOT　SEIZE;

POISONOUS INSECTS do NOT STING him; SAVAGE BEASTS do NOT SEIZE him;

攫　鸟　不　搏；骨　弱　筋　柔　而　握

jué　niǎo　bù　bó;　gǔ　ruò　jīn　róu　ér　wò
GRAB　BIRD　NOT　ATTACK;　BONE　WEAK　MUSCLE　SOFT　BUT　GRASP

固。

gù.
FIRM.

RAPACIOUS BIRDS do NOT ATTACK him; his BONES are WEAK, his MUSCLES are SOFT, BUT his GRASP is FIRM.

未　知　牝　牡　之　合　而　朘　作：

wèi　zhī　pìn　mǔ　zhī　hé　ér　zuī　zuò:
NOT　KNOW　FEMALE　MALE　[PART]　UNION　BUT　CHILD'S-PENIS　ACT:

He has NOT KNOWN the UNION OF FEMALE and MALE, BUT his PENIS becomes ERECT:

精　之　至　也。

jīng　zhī　zhì　yě.
MASCULINE-FORCE　[PART]　EXTREME　[PART].

This results from the ABUNDANCE OF MASCULINE FORCE.

终　日　号　而　不　嗄：

zhōng　rì　háo　ér　bú　shà:
END　DAY　WAIL　BUT　NOT　HOARSE:

Until the END of the DAY he WAILS, BUT he is NOT HOARSE:

和　之　至　也。

hé　　zhī　　zhì　　yě.

HARMONY　[PART]　EXTREME　[PART].

This results from the ABUNDANCE OF HARMONY.

知　和　日　常；知　常　日　明。

zhī　hé　yuē　cháng;　zhī　cháng　yuē　míng.

KNOW　HARMONY　CALL　UNCHANGING;　KNOW　UNCHANGING　CALL　BRIGHT.

To KNOW HARMONY is CALLED "the UNCHANGING;" to KNOW the UNCHANGING is CALLED "BRIGHTNESS."

益　生　日　祥；

yì　　shēng　　yuē　　xiáng;

BENEFIT　LIFE　CALL　INAUSPICIOUS;

To seek BENEFIT in one's own LIFE is CALLED "INAUSPICIOUS;"

心　使　气　日　强。

xīn　shǐ　qì　yuē　qiáng.

HEART　CONTROL　INNER-FORCE　CALL　STRONG.

When the desires of the HEART CONTROL one's INNER FORCE this is CALLED "OVERBEARING."

物　壮　则　老。

wù　　zhuàng　　zé　　lǎo.

THING　STRONG　BUT　OLD.

THINGS may be STRONG, BUT they will become OLD and weak.

谓　之　不　道；不　道　早　已。

wèi　zhī　bú　dào;　bú　dào　zǎo　yǐ.

SAY　THIS　NOT　DAO;　NOT　DAO　EARLY　END.

It is SAID that THIS is NOT the DAO; all things NOT with the DAO meet an EARLY END.

Chapter 56

知　者　不　言；　言　者　不　知。

zhī　　zhě　　bù　　yán;　　yán　　zhě　　bù　　zhī.

KNOW　[PART]　NOT　SPEAK;　SPEAK　[PART]　NOT　KNOW.

Those WHO KNOW do NOT SPEAK; those WHO SPEAK do NOT KNOW.

塞　其　兑；　闭　其　门；

sāi　　qí　　duì;　　bì　　qí　　mén;

STOP-UP　ONE'S　EXCHANGE;　CLOSE　ONE'S　DOOR;

STOP INTERACTING; CLOSE the DOOR;

挫　其　锐；　解　其　纷；

cuò　　qí　　ruì;　　jiě　　qí　　fēn;

BLUNT　ITS　SHARP;　SEPARATE　ITS　ENTANGLED;

BLUNT the SHARP; SEPARATE the ENTANGLED;

和　其　光；　同　其　尘。

huó　　qí　　guāng;　　tóng　　qí　　chén.

DILUTE　ITS　BRIGHT;　UNITE　ITS　DUST.

DILUTE the BRIGHT; UNITE with DUST.

是　谓　玄　同。

shì　　wèi　　xuán　　tóng.

BE　CALL　PROFOUND　UNITY.

This IS CALLED "PROFOUND UNITY."

故　不　可　得　而　亲，　不　可　得　而

gù　　bù　　kě　　dé　　ér　　qīn,　　bù　　kě　　dé　　ér

THEREFORE　NOT　CAN　GAIN　AND　INTIMATE,　NOT　CAN　GAIN　AND

疏；

shū;

DISTANT;

THEREFORE one CANNOT GAIN profound unity AND maintain the notion of INTIMACY, NOR CAN one GAIN it AND maintain the notion of emotional DISTANCE;

不 可 得 而 利， 不 可 得 而 害；

bù   kě   dé   ér   lì,   bù   kě   dé   ér   hài;

NOT   CAN   GAIN   AND   BENEFIT,   NOT   CAN   GAIN   AND   HARM;

One CANNOT GAIN it AND maintain the notion of BENEFIT, NOR CAN one GAIN it AND maintain the notion of HARM;

不 可 得 而 贵， 不 可 得 而 贱。

bù   kě   dé   ér   guì,   bù   kě   dé   ér   jiàn.

NOT   CAN   GAIN   AND   COSTLY,   NOT   CAN   GAIN   AND   HUMBLE.

One CANNOT GAIN it AND maintain the notion of the COSTLY, NOR CAN one GAIN it AND maintain the notion of the HUMBLE.

故 为 天 下 贵。

gù   wéi   tiān   xià   guì.

THUS   BE   HEAVEN   UNDER   HONOR.

THUS it IS HONORED UNDER HEAVEN.

Chapter 57

以　正　治　国；以　奇　用　兵；
yǐ　zhèng　zhì　guó;　yǐ　qí　yòng　bīng;
USE　JUST　RULE　COUNTRY;　USE　SURPRISE　USE　ARMY;

USE JUSTICE in RULING the COUNTRY; USE SURPRISE in DEPLOYING the ARMY;

以　无　事　取　天　下。
yǐ　wú　shì　qǔ　tiān　xià.
TAKE　NOT　AFFAIR　TAKE　HEAVEN　UNDER.

APPLY NON-INTERFERENCE in RULING all things UNDER HEAVEN.

吾　何　以　知　其　然　哉？以　此：
wú　hé　yǐ　zhī　qí　rán　zāi?　yǐ　cǐ:
I　HOW　[PART]　KNOW　THEIR　NATURE　[PART]?　USE　THIS:

HOW do I KNOW the NATURE of THINGS? I USE THIS knowledge:

天　下　多　忌　讳，而　民　弥　贫；
tiān　xià　duō　jì　huì,　ér　mín　mí　pín;
HEAVEN　UNDER　MANY　RESTRICTION,　SO　PEOPLE　MORE　POOR;

When there are MANY RESTRICTIONS UNDER HEAVEN, the PEOPLE become POORER;

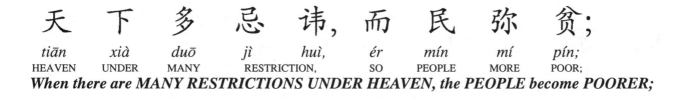

人　多　利　器，国　家　滋　昏；
rén　duō　lì　qì,　guó-　jiā　zī　hūn;
PEOPLE　MANY　SHARP　IMPLEMENT,　COUNTRY-　HOME　MORE　DISORDER;

When the PEOPLE have MANY WEAPONS, the COUNTRY becomes MORE DISORDERED;

人　多　伎　巧，奇　物　滋　起；
rén　duō　jì　qiǎo,　qí　wù　zī　qǐ;
PEOPLE　MORE　TRICKERY　CLEVERNESS,　STRANGE　THING　MORE　OCCUR;

When the PEOPLE exhibit MORE TRICKERY and CLEVERNESS, MORE STRANGE THINGS OCCUR;

法 令 滋 彰, 盗 贼 多 有。

fǎ lìng zī zhāng, dào zéi duō yǒu.

LAW EDICT MORE PROMINENT, BANDIT THIEF MORE EXIST.

When LAWS and EDICTS become MORE PROMINENT, there ARE MORE BANDITS and THIEVES.

故 圣 人 云:

gù shèng- rén yún:

THEREFORE SAGACIOUS- PERSON SAY:

THEREFORE the SAGE SAYS:

我 无 为, 而 民 自 化;

wǒ wú wéi, ér mín zì huà;

I NOT ACT, BUT PEOPLE SELF TRANSFORM;

"I do NOT ACT, BUT the PEOPLE TRANSFORM THEMSELVES;

我 好 静, 而 民 自 正;

wǒ hào jìng, ér mín zì zhèng;

I PREFER TRANQUIL, BUT PEOPLE SELF JUST;

I PREFER TRANQUILITY, BUT the PEOPLE THEMSELVES become JUST;

我 无 事, 而 民 自 富;

wǒ wú shì, ér mín zì fù;

I NOT AFFAIR, BUT PEOPLE SELF WEALTHY;

I do NOT INTERFERE, BUT the PEOPLE THEMSELVES become WEALTHY;

我 无 欲, 而 民 自 朴。

wǒ wú yù, ér mín zì pǔ.

I NOT DESIRE, BUT PEOPLE SELF SIMPLE.

I have NO DESIRES, BUT the PEOPLE THEMSELVES attain SIMPLICITY."

Chapter 58

其　政　闷　闷，　其　民　淳　淳；

qí　zhèng　mèn　mèn,　qí　mín　chún　chún;

ITS　GOVERNMENT　MUFFLED,　ITS　PEOPLE　PURE-AND-SIMPLE;

When the GOVERNMENT is MUFFLED, the PEOPLE are PURE AND SIMPLE;

其　政　察　察，　其　民　缺　缺。

qí　zhèng　chá　chá,　qí　mín　quē　quē.

ITS　GOVERNMENT　CLEVER,　ITS　PEOPLE　FAULT.

When the GOVERNMENT is CLEVER, the PEOPLE develop FAULTS.

祸　兮、福　之　所　倚；

huò　xī,　fú　zhī　suǒ　yǐ;

DISASTER　[PART],　GOOD-FORTUNE　[PART]　WHERE　REST;

As for DISASTER, it is the RESTING PLACE OF GOOD FORTUNE;

福　兮，祸　之　所　伏。

fú　xī,　huò　zhī　suǒ　fú.

GOOD-FORTUNE　[PART],　DISASTER　[PART]　WHERE　HIDE.

As for GOOD FORTUNE, it is the HIDING PLACE OF DISASTER.

孰　知　其　极？其　无　正　也。

shú　zhī　qí　jí?　qí　wú　zhèng　yě.

WHO　KNOW　THEIR　ENDING?　IT　NOT　JUST　[PART].

WHO KNOWS how THINGS will END? THERE is NO JUSTICE.

正　复　为　奇；善　复　为　妖。

zhèng　fù　wéi　qí;　shàn　fù　wéi　yāo.

JUST　RETURN　AS　STRANGE;　GOOD　RETURN　AS　EVIL.

JUSTICE TURNS INTO INJUSTICE; GOOD TURNS INTO EVIL.

人　之　迷，其　日　固　久。

rén　zhī　mí,　qí　rì　gù　jiǔ.

PEOPLE　[PART]　CONFUSION,　ITS　DAY　INDEED　LONG.

As for the PEOPLE'S CONFUSION, ITS DURATION is VERY LONG.

是　以　圣　人　方　而　不　割；廉　而

shì　yǐ　shèng-　rén　fāng　ér　bù　gē;　lián　ér

BE　WHY　SAGACIOUS-　PERSON　SQUARE　BUT　NOT　CUT;　SHARP　BUT

不　刿；

bú　guì;

NOT　STAB;

This is WHY the SAGE is SQUARE BUT does NOT CUT; he is SHARP BUT does NOT STAB;

直　而　不　肆；光　而　不　耀。

zhí　ér　bú　sì;　guāng　ér　bú　yào.

DIRECT　BUT　NOT　UNRESTRAINED;　BRIGHT　BUT　NOT　DAZZLING.

He is DIRECT BUT NOT UNRESTRAINED; he is BRIGHT BUT NOT DAZZLING.

Chapter 59

治　人　事　天，莫　若　啬。
zhì　rén　shì　tiān，　mò　ruò　sè.
GOVERN　PEOPLE　AFFAIR　HEAVEN，　NOT　LIKE　MISERLY.

In GOVERNING the PEOPLE and executing one's DUTIES toward HEAVEN, there is NOTHING LIKE RESTRAINT.

夫　唯　啬，是　谓　早　服。
fú　wéi　sè，　shì　wèi　zǎo　fú.
FOR　MISERLY，　BE　CALL　EARLY　PREPARE.

FOR RESTRAINT IS CALLED "being PREPARED EARLY."

早　服　谓　之　重　积　德。
zǎo　fú　wèi　zhī　chóng　jī　dé.
EARLY　PREPARE　CALL　IT　CONTINUOUSLY ACCUMULATE　VIRTUE.

As for being PREPARED EARLY, one can CALL IT "the CONTINUOUS ACCUMULATION of VIRTUE."

重　积　德　则　无　不　克；
chóng　jī　dé　zé　wú　bú　kè；
CONTINUOUSLY ACCUMULATE　VIRTUE　SO　NOT　NOT　CAN；

When one CONTINUOUSLY ACCUMULATES VIRTUE, there is NOTHING that CANNOT be done;

无　不　克　则　莫　知　其　极；
wú　bú　kè　zé　mò　zhī　qí　jí；
NOT　NOT　CAN　SO　NOT　KNOW　ONE'S　LIMIT；

When there is NOTHING that CANNOT be done, one will KNOW NO LIMITS;

莫　知　其　极，可　以　有　国。
mò　zhī　qí　jí，　kě　yǐ　yǒu　guó.
NOT　KNOW　ONE'S　LIMIT，　CAN　　YI　HAVE　COUNTRY.

If one KNOWS NO LIMITS, one CAN RULE the COUNTRY.

有   国   之   母,   可   以   长   久。

yǒu   *guó*   *zhī*   *mǔ,*   *kě*   *yǐ*   *cháng*   *jiǔ.*

HAVE   COUNTRY   [PART]   MOTHER,   CAN   LONG   LONG-TIME.

If one RULES the COUNTRY in a MOTHERLY way, one CAN LONG CONTINUE.

是   谓   深   根   固   柢。

shì   *wèi*   *shēn*   *gēn*   *gù*   *dǐ.*

BE   SAY   DEEP   ROOT   SOLID   ROOT.

It IS SAID: "DEEP ROOTS, SOLID ROOTS."

长   生   久   视   之   道。

cháng   *shēng*   *jiǔ*   *shì*   *zhī*   *dào.*

LONG   LIFE   LASTING   INSIGHT   [PART]   DAO.

This is the DAO OF LONG LIFE and LASTING INSIGHT.

Chapter 60

治　大　国，　若　烹　小　鲜。

zhì　dà　guó,　ruò　pēng　xiǎo　xiān.
RULE　LARGE　COUNTRY,　LIKE　COOK　SMALL　FISH.

RULING a LARGE COUNTRY is LIKE COOKING a SMALL FISH.

以　道　莅　天　下，　其　鬼　不　神。

yǐ　dào　lì　tiān　xià,　qí　guǐ　bù　shén.
USE　DAO　APPROACH　HEAVEN　UNDER,　ITS　DEMON　NOT　POWER.

USE the DAO to APPROACH all things UNDER HEAVEN, and DEMONS will have NO POWER.

非　其　鬼　不　神，　其　神　不　伤　人。

fēi　qí　guǐ　bù　shén,　qí　shén　bù　shāng　rén.
NOT　ITS　DEMON　NOT　POWER,　THEIR　POWER　NOT　HARM　PERSON.

It is NOT that DEMONS will have NO POWER, but that THEIR POWER will HARM NO ONE.

非　其　神　不　伤　人，

fēi　qí　shén　bù　shāng　rén,
NOT　THEIR　POWER　NOT　HARM　PERSON,

NOT only will THEIR POWER HARM NO ONE,

圣　人　亦　不　伤　人。

shèng-　rén　yì　bù　shāng　rén.
SAGACIOUS-　PERSON　ALSO　NOT　HARM　PERSON.

but the SAGE will ALSO HARM NO ONE.

夫　两　不　相　伤，　故　德　交　归　焉。

fú　liǎng　bù　xiāng　shāng,　gù　dé　jiāo　guī　yān.
FOR　BOTH　NOT　MUTUALLY　HARM,　SO　VIRTUE　MEET　CONVERGE　[PART].

FOR BOTH the sage and the demons MUTUALLY do NO HARM to one another, SO VIRTUE MEETS and CONVERGES.

大　邦　者　下　流;

dà　*bāng*　*zhě*　*xià*　*liú;*
LARGE　COUNTRY　[PART]　LOW　FLOW;

A LARGE COUNTRY is like the LOWER REACHES of a river;

天　下　之　交　也; 天　下　之　牝。

tiān　*xià*　*zhī*　*jiāo*　*yě;*　*tiān*　*xià*　*zhī*　*pìn.*
HEAVEN　UNDER　[PART]　MEET　[PART];　HEAVEN　UNDER　[PART]　FEMININE.

It is the MEETING place OF all things UNDER HEAVEN; it serves as the FEMININE for all things UNDER HEAVEN.

牝　常　以　静　胜　牡;

pìn　*cháng*　*yǐ*　*jìng*　*shèng*　*mǔ;*
FEMININE　ALWAYS　USE　TRANQUIL　OVERCOME　MASCULINE;

The FEMININE ALWAYS USES TRANQUILITY to OVERCOME the MASCULINE;

以　静　为　下。

yǐ　*jìng*　*wéi*　*xià.*
USE　TRANQUIL　ACT　LOW.

It USES TRANQUILITY to ACT with HUMILITY.

故　大　邦　以　下　小　邦,

gù　*dà*　*bāng*　*yǐ*　*xià*　*xiǎo*　*bāng,*
THEREFORE　LARGE　COUNTRY　USE　LOW　SMALL　COUNTRY,

THEREFORE when a LARGE COUNTRY USES HUMILITY toward a SMALL COUNTRY,

则　取　小　邦;

zé　*qǔ*　*xiǎo*　*bāng;*
SO　GAIN　SMALL　COUNTRY;

it GAINS dominion over the SMALL COUNTRY;

小　邦　以　下　大　邦，
xiǎo　bāng　yǐ　xià　dà　bāng,
SMALL　COUNTRY　USE　LOW　LARGE　COUNTRY,

When a SMALL COUNTRY USES HUMILITY toward a LARGE COUNTRY,

则　取　大　邦。
zé　qǔ　dà　bāng.
SO　GAIN　LARGE　COUNTRY.

it GAINS protection from the LARGE COUNTRY.

故　或　下　以　取，或　下　而　取。
gù　huò　xià　yǐ　qǔ,　huò　xià　ér　qǔ.
SO　EITHER　LOW　TO　GAIN,　OR　LOW　AND　GAIN.

SO a country EITHER uses HUMILITY TO GAIN dominion OR it uses HUMILITY AND GAINS protection.

大　邦　不　过　欲　兼　畜　人；
dà　bāng　bú　guò　yù　jiān　xù　rén;
LARGE　COUNTRY　NOT　PASS　DESIRE　SIMULTANEOUSLY　NOURISH　PEOPLE;

A LARGE COUNTRY CANNOT OBVIATE the DESIRE to NOURISH many PEOPLE SIMULTANEOUSLY;

小　邦　不　过　欲　入　事　人。
xiǎo　bāng　bú　guò　yù　rù　shì　rén.
SMALL　COUNTRY　NOT　PASS　DESIRE　ENTER　AFFAIR　PEOPLE.

A SMALL COUNTRY CANNOT OBVIATE the DESIRE to JOIN OTHERS.

夫　两　者，各　得　其　所　欲；
fú　liǎng　zhě,　gè　dé　qí　suǒ　yù;
SO　TWO　[PART],　EACH　GAIN　IT　WHAT　DESIRE;

AS for the TWO countries, EACH GAINS WHAT IT DESIRES;

大　者　宜　为　下。
dà　zhě　yí　wéi　xià.
LARGE　[PART]　FITTING　ACT　LOW.

For the LARGE ONE, it is FITTING to ACT with HUMILITY.

道　者，万　物　之　奥。

dào　zhě,　wàn　wù　zhī　ào.
DAO　[PART], TEN-THOUSAND THING　[PART] PROFOUND.

The DAO is the PROFOUND mystery OF ALL THINGS.

善　人　之　宝；

shàn　rén　zhī　bǎo;
GOOD　PERSON　[PART]　TREASURE;

It is TREASURED by the GOOD PERSON;

不　善　人　之　所　保。

bú　shàn　rén　zhī　suǒ　bǎo.
NOT　GOOD　PERSON　[PART]　WHAT　SAFEGUARD.

It is WHAT is SAFEGUARDED by THOSE who are NOT GOOD.

美　言　可　以　市　尊，

měi　yán　kě　yǐ　shì　zūn;
FINE　SPEECH　CAN　　BUY　HONOR;

FINE SPEECH CAN BUY HONOR;

美　行　可　以　加　人。

měi　xíng　kě　yǐ　jiā　rén.
FINE　DECORUM　CAN　　INCREASE　PERSON.

FINE DECORUM CAN INCREASE a PERSON'S status.

人　之　不　善，何　弃　之　有？

rén　zhī　bú　shàn,　hé　qì　zhī　yǒu?
PERSON　[PART]　NOT　GOOD,　HOW　DISCARD　IT　[PART]?

As for what is NOT GOOD in a PERSON, HOW can one DISCARD IT?

故　立　天　子，　置　三　公，
gù　lì　tiān　zǐ,　zhì　sān　gōng,
THEREFORE ESTABLISH　HEAVEN　SON,　INSTALL　THREE　OFFICIAL,

THEREFORE when ENTHRONING the imperial SON of HEAVEN or INSTALLING the THREE OFFICIALS,

虽　有　拱　璧　以　先　驷　马，
suī　yǒu　gǒng　bì　yǐ　xiān　sì　mǎ,
ALTHOUGH　EXIST　HANDFUL　JADE-BEAD　TAKE　BEFORE　FOUR　HORSE,

ALTHOUGH there ARE HANDFULS of JADE BEADS CARRIED BEFORE a team of FOUR HORSES,

不　如　坐　进　此　道。
bù　rú　zuò-　jìn　cǐ　dào.
NOT　LIKE　SET-　PRESENT　THIS　DAO.

Dealing with these is NOT as FITTING as PRESENTING THIS DAO.

古　之　所　以　贵　此　道　者　何？
gǔ　zhī　suǒ　yǐ　guì　cǐ　dào　zhě　hé?
ANCIENT　[PART]　REASON　HONOR　THIS　DAO　[PART]　WHAT?

Since ANCIENT times, WHAT is the REASON THIS DAO is HONORED?

不　曰：　求　以　得，　有　罪　以　免　邪？
bù　yuē:　qiú　yǐ　dé,　yǒu　zuì　yǐ　miǎn　yé?
NOT　SAY:　SEEK　TAKE　GAIN,　HAVE　GUILT　TAKE　ABSOLVE　[PART]?

Is it NOT SAID: "If you SEEK, you will FIND GAIN; if you HAVE GUILT, you will FIND ABSOLUTION?"

故　为　天　下　贵。
gù　wéi　tiān　xià　guì.
THUS　BE　HEAVEN　UNDER　HONOR.

THUS the dao IS HONORED UNDER HEAVEN.

为　无　为；　事　无　事；　味　无　味。
wéi　wú　wéi;　shì　wú　shì;　wèi　wú　wèi.
ACT　NOT　ACT;　AFFAIR　NOT　AFFAIR;　TASTE　NOT　TASTE.

ENACT NON-ACTION; conduct your AFFAIRS with NON-INTERFERENCE; TASTE what has NO TASTE.

大　小；　多　少；　报　怨　以　德。
dà　xiǎo;　duō　shǎo;　bào　yuàn　yǐ　dé.
BIG　SMALL;　MORE　LESS;　RESPOND　GRIEVANCE　USE　VIRTUE.

BIG is SMALL; MORE is LESS; in RESPONDING to GRIEVANCES USE VIRTUE.

图　难　于　其　易；　为　大　于　其　细。
tú　nán　yú　qí　yì;　wéi　dà　yú　qí　xì.
PURSUE　DIFFICULT　FROM　ITS　EASY;　ACT　GREAT　FROM　ITS　MINUTE.

PURSUE the DIFFICULT FROM the viewpoint of the EASY; ENACT the GREAT FROM the viewpoint of the MINUTE.

天　下　难　事，　必　作　于　易；
tiān　xià　nán　shì,　bì　zuò　yú　yì;
HEAVEN　UNDER　DIFFICULT　AFFAIR,　MUST　DO　FROM　EASY;

UNDER HEAVEN, DIFFICULT AFFAIRS MUST be UNDERTAKEN FROM the viewpoint of the EASY;

天　下　大　事，　必　作　于　细。
tiān　xià　dà　shì,　bì　zuò　yú　xì.
HEAVEN　UNDER　GREAT　AFFAIR,　MUST　DO　FROM　MINUTE.

UNDER HEAVEN, GREAT AFFAIRS MUST be UNDERTAKEN FROM the viewpoint of the MINUTE.

是　以　圣　人　终　不　为　大。
shì　yǐ　shèng-　rén　zhōng　bù　wéi　dà.
BE　WHY　SAGACIOUS-　PERSON　END　NOT　ACT　GREAT.

This IS WHY unto the END of life the SAGE ENACTS no GREAT achievements.

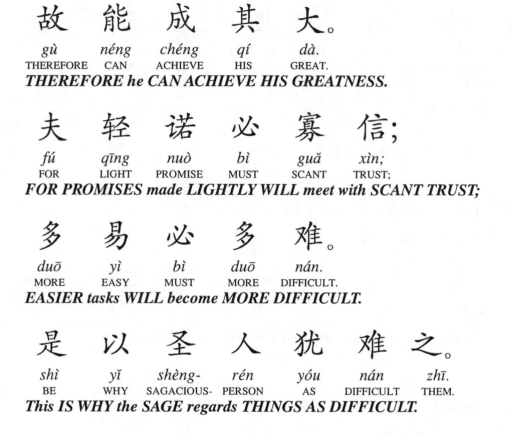

故　能　成　其　大。
gù　néng　chéng　qí　dà.
THEREFORE　CAN　ACHIEVE　HIS　GREAT.

THEREFORE he CAN ACHIEVE HIS GREATNESS.

夫　轻　诺　必　寡　信；
fú　qīng　nuò　bì　guǎ　xìn;
FOR　LIGHT　PROMISE　MUST　SCANT　TRUST;

FOR PROMISES made LIGHTLY WILL meet with SCANT TRUST;

多　易　必　多　难。
duō　yì　bì　duō　nán.
MORE　EASY　MUST　MORE　DIFFICULT.

EASIER tasks WILL become MORE DIFFICULT.

是　以　圣　人　犹　难　之。
shì　yǐ　shèng-　rén　yóu　nán　zhī.
BE　WHY　SAGACIOUS-　PERSON　AS　DIFFICULT　THEM.

This IS WHY the SAGE regards THINGS AS DIFFICULT.

故　终　无　难　矣。
gù　zhōng　wú　nán　yǐ.
THEREFORE　END　NOT　DIFFICULT　[PART].

THEREFORE in the END there are NO DIFFICULTIES.

其　安　易　持;　其　未　兆　易　谋;

qí　ān　yì　chí;　qí　wèi　zhào　yì　móu;

ITS　PEACE　EASY　MAINTAIN;　IT　NOT-YET　PORTEND　EASY　PLAN;

PEACE is EASY to MAINTAIN; WHAT has NOT YET been PORTENDED is EASY to PLAN for;

其　脆　易　泮;　其　微　易　散。

qí　cuì　yì　pàn;　qí　wēi　yì　sàn.

IT　FRAGILE　EASILY　BREAK;　ITS　MINUTE　EASILY　SCATTER.

The FRAGILE is EASILY BROKEN; the MINUTE is EASILY SCATTERED.

为　之　于　未　有;　治　之　于　未　乱。

wéi　zhī　yú　wèi　yǒu;　zhì　zhī　yú　wèi　luàn.

ACT　THEM　FROM　NOT-YET　OCCUR;　CONTROL　THEM　FROM　NOT-YET　DISORDER.

ACT BEFORE things OCCUR; CONTROL THEM BEFORE there is DISORDER.

合　抱　之　木,　生　于　毫　末;

hé　bào　zhī　mù,　shēng　yú　háo　mò;

FIT　EMBRACE　[PART]　TREE,　BORN　FROM　TINY　SHOOT;

A TREE which FITS a person's EMBRACE is BORN FROM a TINY SHOOT;

九　层　之　台,　起　于　累　土;

jiǔ　céng　zhī　tái,　qǐ　yú　lěi　tǔ;

NINE　LEVEL　[PART]　TERRACE,　BEGIN　FROM　PILE　EARTH;

A TERRACE OF NINE LEVELS is BEGUN BY PILING up EARTH;

千　里　之　行,　始　于　足　下。

qiān　lǐ　zhī　xíng,　shǐ　yú　zú　xià.

THOUSAND　LI　[PART]　JOURNEY,　BEGIN　FROM　FOOT　DOWN.

A JOURNEY OF a THOUSAND LI is BEGUN BY putting DOWN one's FOOT.

为　者　败　之；　执　者　失　之。

wéi　zhě　bài　zhī;　zhí　zhě　shī　zhī.

ACT　[PART]　RUIN　THEM;　HOLD　[PART]　LOSE　THEM.

Those WHO ACT on things RUIN THEM; those WHO HOLD to things LOSE THEM.

是　以　圣　人　无　为；　故　无　败；

shì　yí　shèng-　rén　wú　wéi;　gù　wú　bài;

BE　WHY　SAGACIOUS-　PERSON　NOT　ACT;　THEREFORE　NOT　DEFEAT;

This IS WHY the SAGE does NOT ACT; THEREFORE he is NOT DEFEATED;

无　执；　故　无　失。

wú　zhí;　gù　wú　shī.

NOT　HOLD;　THEREFORE　NOT　LOSE.

He does NOT HOLD; THEREFORE he does NOT LOSE.

民　之　从　事，

mín　zhī　cóng　shì,

PEOPLE　[PART]　PURSUE　AFFAIR,

When PEOPLE are PURSUING their AFFAIRS,

常　于　几　成　而　败　之。

cháng　yú　jǐ　chéng　ér　bài　zhī.

ALWAYS　AT　NEARLY　SUCCEED　AND　DEFEAT　THEM.

It is ALWAYS AT the point when they have NEARLY SUCCEEDED that THEY are DEFEATED.

慎　终　如　始，　则　无　败　事。

shèn　zhōng　rú　shǐ,　zé　wú　bài　shì.

CAREFUL　END　AS　BEGINNING,　THEN　NOT　DEFEAT　UNDERTAKING.

If one is as CAREFUL at the END AS at the BEGINNING, THEN one's UNDERTAKINGS will NOT be DEFEATED.

是　以　圣　人　欲　不　欲,

shì　yǐ　shèng-　rén　yù　bú　yù;

BE　WHY　SAGACIOUS-　PERSON　DESIRE　NOT　DESIRE;

This IS WHY the SAGE DESIRES what others do NOT DESIRE;

不　贵　难　得　之　货。

bú　guì　nán　dé　zhī　huò.

NOT　VALUE　DIFFICULT　OBTAIN　[PART]　COMMODITY.

He does NOT VALUE RARE COMMODITIES.

学　不　学;　复　众　人　之　所　过。

xué　bù　xué;　fù　zhòng　rén　zhī　suǒ　guò.

STUDY　NOT　STUDY;　RETURN　NUMEROUS　PERSON　[PART]　WHERE　PASS.

He STUDIES what others do NOT STUDY; he RETURNS WHERE the MULTITUDE have PASSED by.

以　辅　万　物　之　自　然　而　不　敢

yǐ　fǔ　wàn　wù　zhī　zì　rán　ér　bù　gǎn

[PART]　ASSIST　TEN-THOUSAND　THING　[PART]　NATURE　BUT　NOT　DARE

为。

wéi.

ACT.

He ASSISTS ALL THINGS to exist NATURALLY, BUT DARES NOT ACT.

Chapter 65

古　之　善　为　道　者，

gǔ　zhī　shàn　wéi　dào　zhě,

ANCIENT　[PART]　ADEPT　ACT　DAO　[PART],

The ANCIENT ONES ADEPT at ENACTING the DAO

非　以　明　民，　将　以　愚　之。

fēi　yǐ　míng　mín,　jiāng　yǐ　yú　zhī.

NOT　[PART]　ENLIGHTEN　PEOPLE,　TAKE　[PART]　FOOLISH　THEM.

Did NOT ENLIGHTEN the PEOPLE, but LEFT THEM FOOLISH.

民　之　难　治，　以　其　智　多。

mín　zhī　nán　zhì,　yǐ　qí　zhì　duō.

PEOPLE　[PART]　DIFFICULT　GOVERN,　BECAUSE　THEIR　CLEVERNESS　MUCH.

The PEOPLE are DIFFICULT to GOVERN BECAUSE THEY are TOO CLEVER.

故　以　智　治　国，　国　之　贼；

gù　yǐ　zhì　zhì　guó,　guó　zhī　zéi;

THEREFORE　USE　CLEVERNESS　RULE　COUNTRY,　COUNTRY　[PART]　THIEF;

THEREFORE those who USE CLEVERNESS to RULE the COUNTRY are THIEVES with respect to the COUNTRY;

不　以　智　治　国，　国　之　福。

bù　yǐ　zhì　zhì　guó,　guó　zhī　fú.

NOT　USE　CLEVERNESS　RULE　COUNTRY,　COUNTRY　[PART] GOOD-FORTUNE.

Those who do NOT USE CLEVERNESS to RULE the COUNTRY are the GOOD FORTUNE OF the COUNTRY.

知　此　两　者，　亦　稽　式。

zhī　cǐ　liǎng　zhě,　yì　jī　shì.

KNOW　THESE　TWO　[PART],　ALSO　ASSESS　METHOD.

KNOWING THESE TWO precepts is ALSO the way to ASSESS one's METHOD.

常　知　稽　式，　是　谓　玄　德。

cháng　zhī　jī　shì,　shì　wèi　xuán　dé.

ALWAYS　KNOW　ASSESS　METHOD,　BE　CALL　PROFOUND　VIRTUE.

ALWAYS KNOWING how to ASSESS one's METHOD IS CALLED "PROFOUND VIRTUE."

玄　德　深　矣；　远　矣；　与　物　反　矣。

xuán　dé　shēn　yǐ;　yuǎn　yǐ;　yǔ　wù　fǎn　yǐ.

PROFOUND　VIRTUE　DEEP　[PART];　FAR　[PART];　HELP　THING　RETURN　[PART].

PROFOUND VIRTUE is DEEP; it goes FAR; it HELPS all THINGS RETURN to the dao.

然　后　乃　至　大　顺。

rán　hòu　nǎi　zhì　dà　shùn.

[PART]　AFTER　BE　TO　GREAT　SUBMISSION.

THEN this LEADS TO GREAT SUBMISSION.

Chapter 66

江　海　之　所　以　能　为　百　谷　王，

jiāng　*hǎi*　*zhī*　*suǒ*　*yǐ*　*néng*　*wéi*　*bǎi*　*gǔ*　*wáng,*

RIVER　OCEAN　[PART]　REASON　　CAN　ACT　HUNDRED　VALLEY　KING,

The REASON great RIVERS and OCEANS CAN ACT as KING of a HUNDRED river VALLEYS

以　其　善　下　之；　故　能　为　百　谷

yǐ　*qí*　*shàn*　*xià*　*zhī;*　*gù*　*néng*　*wéi*　*bǎi*　*gǔ*

TAKE　THEY　ADEPT　BELOW　THEM;　THEREFORE　CAN　ACT　HUNDRED　VALLEY

王。

wáng.

KING.

IS that THEY are ADEPT at lying BELOW the VALLEYS; THEREFORE they CAN ACT as KING of a HUNDRED VALLEYS.

是　以　圣　人　欲　上　民，

shì　*yǐ*　*shèng-*　*rén*　*yù*　*shàng*　*mín,*

BE　WHY　SAGACIOUS-　PERSON　DESIRE　ABOVE　PEOPLE,

This IS WHY the SAGE who DESIRES to be ABOVE the PEOPLE

必　以　言　下　之；

bì　*yǐ*　*yán*　*xià*　*zhī;*

MUST　USE　SPEECH　BELOW　THEM;

MUST SPEAK as if he were BELOW THEM;

欲　先　民，　必　以　身　后　之。

yù　*xiān*　*mín,*　*bì*　*yǐ*　*shēn*　*hòu*　*zhī.*

DESIRE　BEFORE　PEOPLE,　MUST　TAKE　BODY　BEHIND　THEM.

If he DESIRES to be BEFORE the PEOPLE, he MUST PLACE HIMSELF BEHIND THEM.

是　以　圣　人　处　上，　而　民　不　重；

shì　*yǐ*　*shèng-*　*rén*　*chǔ*　*shàng,*　*ér*　*mín*　*bú*　*zhòng;*

BE　WHY　SAGACIOUS-　PERSON　OCCUPY　ABOVE,　WHEREAS　PEOPLE　NOT　HEAVY;

This IS WHY the SAGE IS ABOVE, WHEREAS the PEOPLE do NOT find his rulership HEAVY;

处　前，　而　民　不　害。

chǔ　*qián,*　*ér*　*mín*　*bú*　*hài.*
OCCUPY　BEFORE,　BUT　PEOPLE　NOT　HARM.

He IS BEFORE, BUT the PEOPLE are NOT HARMED.

是　以　天　下　乐　推　而　不　厌。

shì　*yǐ*　*tiān*　*xià*　*lè*　*tuī*　*ér*　*bú*　*yàn.*
BE　WHY　HEAVEN　UNDER　GLADLY　SUPPORT　AND　NOT　DESPISE.

This IS WHY all things UNDER HEAVEN GLADLY SUPPORT him AND do NOT DESPISE him.

以　其　不　争，　故　天　下　莫　能　与

yǐ　*qí*　*bù*　*zhēng,*　*gù*　*tiān*　*xià*　*mò*　*néng*　*yǔ*
SINCE　HE　NOT　CONTEND,　SO　HEAVEN　UNDER　NOT　CAN　WITH

之　争。

zhī　*zhēng.*
HIM　CONTEND.

SINCE HE does NOT CONTEND, NOTHING UNDER HEAVEN CAN CONTEND WITH HIM.

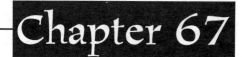

Chapter 67

天　下　皆　谓　我　道　大；似　不　肖。

tiān　xià　jiē　wèi　wǒ　dào　dà;　sì　bú　xiào.

HEAVEN　UNDER　ALL　SAY　MY　DAO　GREAT;　SEEM　NOT　RESEMBLE.

UNDER HEAVEN, EVERYONE SAYS that MY DAO is GREAT; it SEEMS to RESEMBLE NOTHING else.

夫　唯　大，故　似　不　肖。

fú　wéi　dà,　gù　sì　bú　xiào.

SINCE　GREAT,　SO　SEEM　NOT　RESEMBLE.

SINCE it is GREAT, it SEEMS to RESEMBLE NOTHING else.

若　肖，久　矣　其　细　也　夫。

ruò　xiào,　jiǔ　yǐ　qí　xì　yě　fú.

IF　RESEMBLE,　LONG　[PART]　IT　TRIFLING　[PART]　[PART].

IF it RESEMBLED anything, IT would LONG ago have become a TRIFLING thing.

我　有　三　宝，持　而　保　之：

wǒ　yǒu　sān　bǎo,　chí　ér　bǎo　zhī:

I　HAVE　THREE　TREASURE,　MAINTAIN　AND　SAFEGUARD　THEM:

I HAVE THREE TREASURES; I MAINTAIN AND SAFEGUARD THEM:

一　日　慈；二　日　俭；

yī　yuē　cí;　èr　yuē　jiǎn;

ONE　CALL　KINDNESS;　TWO　CALL　FRUGAL;

The FIRST is CALLED "KINDNESS;" the SECOND is CALLED "FRUGALITY;"

三　日　不　敢　为　天　下　先。

sān　yuē　bù　gǎn　wéi　tiān　xià　xiān.

THREE　CALL　NOT　DARE　ACT　HEAVEN　UNDER　FIRST.

The THIRD is CALLED "NOT DARING to ACT as the FIRST UNDER HEAVEN."

慈　故　能　勇；

cí　gù　néng　yǒng;

KINDNESS　SO　CAN　BRAVE;

If one has KINDNESS, one CAN be BRAVE;

俭　　故　　能　　广;

jiǎn　　*gù*　　*néng*　　*guǎng;*
FRUGAL　　SO　　CAN　　VAST;

If one is FRUGAL, one CAN be VAST;

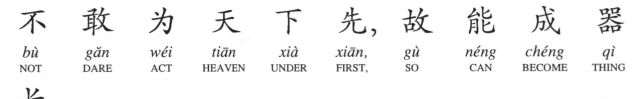

不　　敢　　为　　天　　下　　先,　　故　　能　　成　　器

bù　　*gǎn*　　*wéi*　　*tiān*　　*xià*　　*xiān,*　　*gù*　　*néng*　　*chéng*　　*qì*
NOT　　DARE　　ACT　　HEAVEN　　UNDER　　FIRST,　　SO　　CAN　　BECOME　　THING

长。

zhǎng.
RULER.

If one DARES NOT ACT as the FIRST UNDER HEAVEN, one CAN BECOME RULER of all THINGS.

今　　舍　　慈　　且　　勇;　　舍　　俭　　且　　广;

jīn　　*shě*　　*cí*　　*qiě*　　*yǒng;*　　*shě*　　*jiǎn*　　*qiě*　　*guǎng;*
TODAY　　ABANDON　　KINDNESS　　BUT　　BRAVE;　　ABANDON　　FRUGAL　　BUT　　VAST;

TODAY people ABANDON KINDNESS, BUT act BRAVE; they ABANDON FRUGALITY, BUT act VAST;

舍　　后　　且　　先;　　死　　矣。

shě　　*hòu*　　*qiě*　　*xiān;*　　*sǐ*　　*yǐ.*
ABANDON　　BEHIND　　BUT　　FIRST;　　DEATH　　[PART].

They ABANDON placing themselves BEHIND, BUT place themselves FIRST; this is DEATH.

夫　　慈,　　以　　战　　则　　胜;　　以　　守　　则　　固。

fú　　*cí,*　　*yǐ*　　*zhàn*　　*zé*　　*shèng;*　　*yǐ*　　*shǒu*　　*zé*　　*gù.*
FOR　　KINDNESS,　　TAKE　　BATTLE　　SO　　WIN;　　TAKE　　DEFEND　　SO　　SOLID.

FOR if KINDNESS TAKES up the BATTLE, the battle will be WON; if kindness TAKES up the DEFENSE, the defense will be SOLID.

天　　将　　救　　之,　　以　　慈　　卫　　之。

tiān　　*jiāng*　　*jiù*　　*zhī,*　　*yǐ*　　*cí*　　*wèi*　　*zhī.*
HEAVEN　　FUTURE　　SAVE　　THEM,　　USE　　KINDNESS　　PROTECT　　THEM.

When HEAVEN SAVES all THINGS, it will USE KINDNESS to PROTECT THEM.

Chapter 68

善 为 士 者， 不 武；
shàn *wéi* *shì* *zhě,* *bù* *wǔ;*
ADEPT BE SOLDIER [PART], NOT MARTIAL-ART;
Those WHO are ADEPT at BEING SOLDIERS use NO MARTIAL ARTS;

善 战 者， 不 怒；
shàn *zhàn* *zhě,* *bú* *nù;*
ADEPT BATTLE [PART], NOT ANGER;
Those WHO are ADEPT at doing BATTLE have NO ANGER;

善 胜 敌 者， 不 与；
shàn *shèng* *dí* *zhě,* *bú* *yù;*
ADEPT OVERCOME ENEMY [PART], NOT PARTICIPATE;
Those WHO are ADEPT at OVERCOMING the ENEMY do NOT PARTICIPATE in battle;

善 用 人 者， 为 之 下。
shàn *yòng* *rén* *zhě,* *wéi* *zhī* *xià.*
ADEPT USE PERSON [PART], ACT [PART] BELOW.
Those WHO are ADEPT at ADMINISTRATING ACT HUMBLE.

是 谓 不 争 之 德；
shì *wèi* *bù* *zhēng* *zhī* *dé;*
BE CALL NOT CONTEND [PART] VIRTUE;
This IS CALLED "the VIRTUE of NOT CONTENDING;"

是 谓 用 人 之 力；
shì *wèi* *yòng* *rén* *zhī* *lì;*
BE CALL USE PERSON [PART] ABILITY;
This IS CALLED "the ABILITY to ADMINISTRATE;"

是 谓 配 天 古 之 极。
shì *wèi* *pèi* *tiān* *gǔ* *zhī* *jí.*
BE CALL JOIN HEAVEN ANCIENT [PART] LIMIT.
This IS CALLED "JOINING with the ANCIENT LIMIT of HEAVEN."

Chapter 69

用　兵　有　言:

yòng　bīng　yǒu　yán:

USE　MILITARY-FORCE　EXIST　SAYING:

As for the USE of MILITARY FORCE, there IS a SAYING:

吾　不　敢　为　主,　而　为　客;

wú　bù　gǎn　wéi　zhǔ,　ér　wéi　kè;

I　NOT　DARE　ACT　HOST,　BUT　ACT　GUEST;

"I DARE NOT ACT as HOST, BUT I will ACT as a GUEST;

不　敢　进　寸,　而　退　尺。

bù　gǎn　jìn　cún,　ér　tuì　chǐ.

NOT　DARE　ADVANCE　INCH,　BUT　RETREAT　FOOT.

I DARE NOT ADVANCE one INCH, BUT I will RETREAT one FOOT."

是　谓　行　无　行;　攘　无　臂;

shì　wèi　xíng　wú　xíng;　rǎng　wú　bì;

BE　CALL　MOVE　NOT　MOVE;　PUSH-UP-SLEEVES　NOT　ARM;

This IS CALLED "MOVING WITHOUT MOVING; PUSHING UP ONE'S SLEEVES WITHOUT baring one's ARMS;

扔　无　敌;　执　无　兵。

rēng　wú　dí;　zhí　wú　bīng.

CAST　NOT　ENEMY;　HOLD　NOT　WEAPON.

CASTING one's weapon WITHOUT an ENEMY; HOLDING on WITHOUT a WEAPON."

祸　莫　大　于　轻　敌;

huò　mò　dà　yú　qīng　dí;

DISASTER　NOT　GREATER　THAN　LIGHTLY　ENEMY;

There is NO GREATER DISASTER THAN taking the ENEMY LIGHTLY;

轻　敌　几　丧　吾　宝。
qīng　dí　jǐ　sāng　wú　bǎo.
LIGHTLY　ENEMY　NEARLY　LOSE　MY　TREASURE.
If I take the ENEMY LIGHTLY I will come CLOSE to LOSING MY TREASURES.

故　抗　兵　相　若；哀　者　胜　矣。
gù　kàng　bīng　xiāng　ruò；　āi　zhě　shèng　yǐ.
ENEMY　RESIST　ARMY　MUTUALLY　SIMILAR；　GRIEF　[PART]　VICTORY　[PART].
When RESISTING the ENEMY, the ARMIES are MUTUALLY SIMILAR; the side that is GRIEVING will gain VICTORY.

吾　言　甚　易　知，　甚　易　行。

wú　yán　shèn　yì　zhī,　shèn　yì　xíng.
MY　WORD　VERY　EASY　KNOW,　VERY　EASY　APPLY.

MY WORDS are VERY EASY to UNDERSTAND and VERY EASY to APPLY.

天　下　莫　能　知，　莫　能　行。

tiān　xià　mò　néng　zhī,　mò　néng　xíng.
HEAVEN　UNDER　NOT　CAN　KNOW,　NOT　CAN　APPLY.

Yet UNDER HEAVEN NO ONE CAN UNDERSTAND them and NO ONE CAN APPLY them.

言　有　宗；　事　有　君。

yán　yǒu　zōng;　shì　yǒu　jūn.
WORD　HAVE　MASTER;　AFFAIR　HAVE　SOVEREIGN.

My WORDS HAVE a MASTER; my AFFAIRS HAVE a SOVEREIGN.

夫　唯　无　知，　是　以　不　我　知。

fú　wéi　wú　zhī,　shì　yǐ　bù　wǒ　zhī.
　　SINCE　NOT　KNOW,　BE　WHY　NOT　ME　KNOW.

SINCE people do NOT UNDERSTAND my words, they do NOT UNDERSTAND ME.

知　我　者　希；　则　我　者　贵。

zhī　wǒ　zhě　xī,　zé　wǒ　zhě　guì.
KNOW　ME　[PART]　FEW;　FOLLOW　ME　[PART]　PRECIOUS.

Those WHO UNDERSTAND ME are FEW; those WHO FOLLOW ME are RARE.

是　以　圣　人　被　褐　而　怀　玉。

shì　yǐ　shèng-　rén　bèi　hè　ér　huái　yù.
BE　WHY　SAGACIOUS-　PERSON　WEAR　COARSE-CLOTH　BUT　HOLD　JADE.

This IS WHY the SAGE WEARS COARSE CLOTH BUT HOLDS JADE.

知　不　知，尚　矣；
zhī　bù　zhī，shàng　yǐ;
KNOW　NOT　KNOW，ESTEEMED　[PART];

To KNOW that one does NOT KNOW is BEST;

不　知　知，病　也。
bù　zhī　zhī，bìng　yě.
NOT　KNOW　KNOW，SHORTCOMING　[PART].

NOT to KNOW that one KNOWS is a SHORTCOMING.

圣　人　不　病，
shèng-　rén　bú　bìng,
SAGACIOUS-　PERSON　NOT　SHORTCOMING,

The SAGE has NO SHORTCOMINGS

以　其　病　病。
yǐ　qí　bìng　bìng.
BECAUSE　HIS　SHORTCOMING　SHORTCOMING.

BECAUSE he acknowledges HIS SHORTCOMINGS as SHORTCOMINGS.

夫　唯　病　病，是　以　不　病。
fú　wéi　bìng　bìng，shì　yǐ　bú　bìng.
SINCE　SHORTCOMING SHORTCOMING，BE　WHY　NOT　SHORTCOMING.

SINCE he acknowledges his SHORTCOMINGS as SHORTCOMINGS, he has NO SHORTCOMINGS.

民　不　畏　威，　则　大　威　至。

mín　bú　wèi　wēi,　zé　dà　wēi　zhì.

PEOPLE　NOT　FEAR　FORCE,　THEN　GREAT　CALAMITY　ARRIVE.

When the PEOPLE FEAR NO FORCE, THEN GREAT CALAMITY will ARRIVE.

无　狎　其　所　居；

wú　xiá　qí　suǒ　jū;

NOT　FORCE　THEIR　[PART]　DWELLING;

Do NOT FORCE your way into THEIR DWELLINGS;

无　厌　其　所　生。

wú　yàn　qí　suǒ　shēng.

NOT　DETEST　THEIR　[PART]　LIVELIHOOD.

Do NOT DETEST THEIR means of LIVELIHOOD.

夫　唯　不　厌，　是　以　不　厌。

fú　wéi　bú　yàn,　shì　yǐ　bú　yàn.

FOR　NOT　DETEST,　BE　WHY　NOT　DETEST.

FOR if the ruler does NOT DETEST the people, the people will NOT DETEST the ruler.

是　以　圣　人　自　知，　不　自　见；

shì　yǐ　shèng-　rén　zì　zhī,　bú　zì　xiàn;

BE　WHY　SAGACIOUS-　PERSON　SELF　KNOW,　NOT　SELF　SHOW;

This IS WHY the SAGE KNOWS HIMSELF but does NOT SHOW HIMSELF;

自　爱，　不　自　贵。

zì　ài,　bú　zì　guì.

SELF　RESPECT,　NOT　SELF　HONOR.

He RESPECTS HIMSELF, but does NOT make a show of HONORING HIMSELF.

故　去　彼　取　此。

gù　qù　bǐ　qǔ　cǐ.

THEREFORE　GO　THAT　TAKE　THIS.

THEREFORE he LEAVES THAT and TAKES THIS.

Chapter 73

勇 于 敢 则 杀;

yǒng *yú* *gǎn* *zé* *shā;*
BRAVE AND DARE SO KILL;

Those who are BRAVE AND IMPETUOUS will be KILLED;

勇 于 不 敢 则 活。

yǒng *yú* *bù* *gǎn* *zé* *huó.*
BRAVE BUT NOT DARE SO LIVE.

Those who are BRAVE BUT NOT IMPETUOUS will LIVE.

此 两 者, 或 利 或 害。

cǐ *liǎng* *zhě,* *huò* *lì* *huò* *hài.*
THESE TWO [PART], EITHER BENEFIT OR HARM.

Of THESE TWO, ONE brings BENEFIT and the OTHER brings HARM.

天 之 所 恶, 孰 知 其 故?

tiān *zhī* *suǒ* *wù,* *shú* *zhī* *qí* *gù?*
HEAVEN [PART] WHAT DETEST, WHO KNOW ITS REASON?

As for WHAT HEAVEN DETESTS, WHO KNOWS the REASON?

是 以 圣 人 犹 难 之。

shì *yǐ* *shèng-* *rén* *yóu* *nán* *zhī.*
BE WHY SAGACIOUS- PERSON SEEM DIFFICULT IT.

This IS WHY even the SAGE SEEMS to find THIS question DIFFICULT.

天 之 道, 不 争 而 善 胜;

tiān *zhī* *dào,* *bù* *zhēng* *ér* *shàn* *shèng;*
HEAVEN [PART] DAO, NOT CONTEND BUT ADEPT VICTORY;

The DAO of HEAVEN does NOT CONTEND, BUT ADEPTLY gains VICTORY;

不　言　而　善　应；　不　召　而　自　来；
bù　yán　ér　shàn　yìng;　bú　zhào　ér　zì　lái;
NOT　SPEAK　BUT　ADEPT　ANSWER;　NOT　SUMMON　BUT　SELF　COME;

It does NOT SPEAK, BUT ADEPTLY ANSWERS; it does NOT SUMMON, BUT all things WILLINGLY COME;

绰　然　而　善　谋。
chán　rán　ér　shàn　móu.
　CALM　BUT　ADEPT　PLAN.

It is CALM, BUT ADEPT at PLANNING.

天　网　恢　恢；　疏　而　不　失。
tiān　wǎng　huī　huī;　shū　ér　bù　shī.
HEAVEN　NET　VAST;　SPARSE　BUT　NOT　LOSE.

The NET of HEAVEN is VAST; its mesh is SPARSE BUT it NEVER LOSES its catch.

Chapter 74

民 不 畏 死 , 奈 何 以 死 惧 之 ?

mín *bú* *wèi* *sǐ,* *nài* *hé* *yǐ* *sǐ* *jù* *zhī?*

PEOPLE NOT FEAR DEATH, HOW USE DEATH FRIGHTEN THEM?

If the PEOPLE do NOT FEAR DEATH, HOW can the ruler USE DEATH to INTIMIDATE THEM?

若 使 民 常 畏 死 , 而 为 奇 者 ,

ruò *shǐ* *mín* *cháng* *wèi* *sǐ,* *ér* *wéi* *qí* *zhě,*

IF CAUSE PEOPLE ALWAYS FEAR DEATH, SO ACT STRANGELY [PART],

IF the ruler ENSURES that the PEOPLE ALWAYS FEAR DEATH, as for those WHO ACT CRIMINALLY,

吾 得 执 而 杀 之 , 孰 敢 ?

wú *dé* *zhí* *ér* *shā* *zhī,* *shú* *gǎn?*

I GAIN SEIZE AND KILL THEM, WHO DARE?

If I TAKE them, SEIZE them AND KILL THEM, WHO will DARE to act criminally?

常 有 司 杀 者 杀 。

cháng *yǒu* *sī* *shā* *zhě* *shā.*

ALWAYS EXIST ATTEND KILL [PART] KILL.

There IS ALWAYS an EXECUTIONER to do the KILLING.

夫 代 司 杀 者 杀 ,

fú *dài* *sī* *shā* *zhě* *shā,*

FOR TAKE-PLACE-OF ATTEND KILL [PART] KILL,

FOR TAKING the PLACE OF the EXECUTIONER and KILLING

是 谓 代 大 匠 斲 。

shì *wèi* *dài* *dà* *jiàng* *zhuó.*

BE CALL TAKE-PLACE-OF GREAT CRAFTSMAN CHOP.

IS CALLED "TAKING the PLACE OF the GREAT CRAFTSMAN at WOODWORKING."

夫　代　大　匠　斲　者，

fú　*dài*　*dà*　*jiàng*　*zhuó*　*zhě*,

FOR　TAKE-PLACE-OF　GREAT　CRAFTSMAN　CHOP　[PART],

As for those WHO TAKE the PLACE OF the GREAT CRAFTSMAN at WOODWORKING,

希　有　不　伤　其　手　者　矣。

xī　*yǒu*　*bù*　*shāng*　*qí*　*shǒu*　*zhě*　*yǐ*.

FEW　EXIST　NOT　INJURE　THEIR　HAND　[PART]　[PART].

There ARE FEW WHO AVOID INJURING THEIR HANDS.

Chapter 75

民　之　饥，　以　其　上　食　税　之　多；
mín　zhī　jǐ,　yǐ　qí　shàng　shí　shuì　zhī　duō;
PEOPLE　[PART]　HUNGER,　BECAUSE　THEIR　RULER　EAT　TAX　[PART]　MANY;

The PEOPLE are HUNGRY BECAUSE the RULER DEVOURS too MANY TAXES;

是　以　饥。
shì　yǐ　jǐ.
BE　WHY　HUNGER.

This IS WHY there is HUNGER.

民　之　难　治，　以　其　上　之　有　为；
mín　zhī　nán　zhì,　yǐ　qí　shàng　zhī　yǒu　wéi;
PEOPLE　[PART]　DIFFICULT　GOVERN,　BECAUSE　THEIR　RULE　IT　HAVE　ACT;

The PEOPLE are DIFFICULT to GOVERN BECAUSE the RULER ACTS;

是　以　难　治。
shì　yǐ　nán　zhì.
BE　WHY　DIFFICULT　GOVERN.

This IS WHY the people are DIFFICULT to GOVERN.

民　之　轻　死，
mín　zhī　qīng　sǐ,
PEOPLE　[PART]　LIGHTLY　DIE,

PEOPLE take DEATH LIGHTLY

以　其　上　求　生　之　厚；
yǐ　qí　shàng　qiú　shēng　zhī　hòu;
BECAUSE　THEIR　RULER　DEMAND　LIFE　[PART]　THICK;

BECAUSE the RULER DEMANDS too MUCH of LIFE;

是　以　轻　死。

shì　*yǐ*　*qīng*　*sǐ*.

BE　WHY　LIGHTLY　DIE.

This IS WHY the people take DEATH LIGHTLY.

夫　唯　无　以　生　为　者，

fú　*wéi*　*wú*　*yǐ*　*shēng*　*wéi*　*zhě*,

FOR　NOT　USE　LIFE　ACT　[PART],

FOR those WHO do NOT USE their LIFE to ACT

是　贤　于　贵　生。

shì　*xián*　*yú*　*guì*　*shēng*.

BE　ABLE　AT　VALUE　LIFE.

ARE ABLE TO VALUE LIFE.

Chapter 76

人　之　生　也　柔　弱；

rén　zhī　shēng　yě　róu　ruò;

PEOPLE　[PART]　LIVE　[PART]　SOFT　WEAK;

While PEOPLE LIVE, their bodies are SOFT and WEAK;

其　死　也　堅　強。

qí　sǐ　yě　jiān　qiáng.

THEIR　DEATH　[PART]　HARD　STIFF.

Upon THEIR DEATH, they are HARD and STIFF.

草　木　之　生　也　柔　脆；

cǎo　mù　zhī　shēng　yě　róu　cuì;

GRASS　TREE　[PART]　LIVE　[PART]　SOFT　FRAGILE;

While GRASSES and TREES LIVE, they are SOFT and FRAGILE;

其　死　也　枯　槁。

qí　sǐ　yě　kū　gǎo.

THEIR　DEATH　[PART]　WITHERED　STALK.

Upon THEIR DEATH they are WITHERED STALKS.

故　堅　強　者　死　之　徒；

gù　jiān　qiáng　zhě　sǐ　zhī　tú;

THEREFORE　HARD　STIFF　[PART]　DEATH　[PART]　FOLLOWER;

THEREFORE the HARD and STIFF are the FOLLOWERS of DEATH;

柔　弱　者　生　之　徒。

róu　ruò　zhě　shēng　zhī　tú.

SOFT　WEAK　[PART]　LIFE　[PART]　FOLLOWER.

The SOFT and WEAK are the FOLLOWERS of LIFE.

是　以　兵　强　则　灭；木　强　则　折。

shì　　yǐ　　bīng　qiáng　　zé　　miè;　　mù　　qiáng　　zé　　zhé.
BE　　WHY　ARMY　STRONG　YET　ANNIHILATE;　TREE　STRONG　YET　SNAP.

This IS WHY an ARMY may be STRONG, YET be ANNIHILATED; a TREE may be STRONG, YET its branches can be SNAPPED off.

坚　强　处　下；柔　弱　处　上。

jiān　qiáng　chǔ　xià;　róu　ruò　chǔ　shàng.
HARD　STIFF　OCCUPY　INFERIOR;　SOFT　WEAK　OCCUPY　SUPERIOR.

The HARD and STIFF ARE INFERIOR; the SOFT and WEAK ARE SUPERIOR.

Chapter 77

天　之　道，其　犹　张　弓　欤？

tiān　zhī　dào,　qí　yóu　zhāng　gōng　yú?
HEAVEN　[PART]　DAO,　IT　LIKE　STRETCH　BOW　[PART]?

As for the DAO OF HEAVEN, is IT not LIKE STRETCHING a BOW?

高　者　抑　之；下　者　举　之；

gāo　zhě　yì　zhī;　xià　zhě　jǔ　zhī;
HIGH　[PART]　RESTRAIN　IT;　LOW　[PART]　RAISE　IT;

If the bow is too HIGH IT is LOWERED; if it is too LOW IT is RAISED;

有　馀　者　损　之；

yǒu　yú　zhě　sǔn　zhī;
EXIST　EXCESS　[PART]　DECREASE　IT;

If the tension is EXCESSIVE, IT is DECREASED;

不　足　者　补　之。

bù　zú　zhě　bǔ　zhī.
NOT　SUFFICIENT　[PART]　SUPPLEMENT　IT.

If INSUFFICIENT, IT is SUPPLEMENTED.

天　之　道，

tiān　zhī　dào,
HEAVEN　[PART]　DAO,

The DAO of HEAVEN

损　有　馀　而　补　不　足。

sǔn　yǒu　yú　ér　bǔ　bù　zú.
DECREASE　EXIST　EXCESS　AND　SUPPLEMENT　NOT　SUFFICIENT.

Is to DECREASE the EXCESSIVE AND SUPPLEMENT the INSUFFICIENT.

人　之　道，則　不　然：

rén　zhī　dào,　zé　bù　rán:

MANKIND　[PART]　DAO,　BUT　NOT　THUS:

BUT the DAO of MANKIND is NOT THUS:

损　不　足　以　奉　有　馀。

sǔn　bù　zú　yǐ　fèng　yǒu　yú.

DECREASE　NOT　SUFFICIENT　TO　PRESENT　EXIST　EXCESS.

It DECREASES the INSUFFICIENT TO PRESENT it where there IS EXCESS.

孰　能　有　馀　以　奉　天　下？

shú　néng　yǒu　yú　yǐ　fèng　tiān　xià?

WHO　CAN　HAVE　EXCESS　[PART]　PRESENT　HEAVEN　UNDER?

WHO CAN TAKE the EXCESS and PRESENT it to all things UNDER HEAVEN?

唯　有　道　者。

wéi　yǒu　dào　zhě.

ONLY　HAVE　DAO　[PART].

ONLY those WHO HAVE the DAO.

是　以　圣　人　为　而　不　恃；

shì　yǐ　shèng-　rén　wéi　ér　bú　shì;

BE　WHY　SAGACIOUS-　PERSON　ACT　BUT　NOT　DEPEND;

This IS WHY the SAGE ACTS BUT does NOT DEPEND;

功　成　而　不　处；

gōng　chéng　ér　bù　chǔ;

MERITORIOUS-ACT　ACCOMPLISH　BUT　NOT　DWELL;

He ACCOMPLISHES MERITORIOUS ACTS BUT does NOT DWELL on them;

其　不　欲　见　贤。

qí　bú　yù　jiàn　xián.

HE　NOT　DESIRE　SHOW　VIRTUE.

HE has NO DESIRE to SHOW his VIRTUE.

Chapter 78

天　下　莫　柔　弱　于　水，

tiān　*xià*　*mò*　*róu*　*ruò*　*yú*　*shuǐ,*

HEAVEN　UNDER　NOT　SOFT　WEAK　THAN　WATER,

UNDER HEAVEN there is NOTHING SOFTER and WEAKER THAN WATER,

而　攻　坚　强　者　莫　之　能　胜；

ér　*gōng*　*jiān*　*qiáng*　*zhě*　*mò*　*zhī*　*néng*　*shèng;*

YET　ATTACK　HARD　STIFF　[PART]　NOT　IT　CAN　SURPASS;

YET for ATTACKING the HARD and STIFF, NOTHING CAN SURPASS IT;

以　其　无　以　易　之。

yǐ　*qí*　*wú*　*yǐ*　*yì*　*zhī.*

BECAUSE　IT　NOT　[PART]　EASY　IT.

This is BECAUSE there is NOTHING that can EASILY replace IT.

弱　之　胜　强；柔　之　胜　刚。

ruò　*zhī*　*shèng*　*qiáng;*　*róu*　*zhī*　*shèng*　*gāng.*

WEAK　[PART]　CONQUER　STRONG;　SOFT　[PART]　CONQUER　HARD.

The WEAK CONQUERS the STRONG; the SOFT CONQUERS the HARD.

天　下　莫　不　知，莫　能　行。

tiān　*xià*　*mò*　*bù*　*zhī,*　*mò*　*néng*　*xíng.*

HEAVEN　UNDER　NOT　NOT　KNOW,　NOT　CAN　APPLY.

UNDER HEAVEN there is NO ONE who does NOT KNOW this, yet NO ONE CAN APPLY this.

是　以　圣　人　云：

shì　*yǐ*　*shèng-*　*rén*　*yún:*

BE　WHY　SAGACIOUS-　PERSON　SAY:

This IS WHY the SAGE SAYS:

受 国 之 垢, 是 谓 社 稷 主;

shòu   *guó*   *zhī*   *gòu,*   *shì*   *wèi*   *shè*   *jì*   *zhǔ;*

RECEIVE   COUNTRY   [PART]   HUMILIATION,   BE   CALL   STATE   MASTER;

"He who TAKES on the HUMILIATIONS OF the COUNTRY IS CALLED MASTER of the STATE;

受 国 不 祥, 是 为 天 下 王。

shòu   *guó*   *bù*   *xiáng,*   *shì*   *wéi*   *tiān*   *xià*   *wáng.*

RECEIVE   COUNTRY   NOT   AUSPICIOUS,   BE   ACT   HEAVEN   UNDER   KING.

He who TAKES on the MISFORTUNES of the COUNTRY ACTS as KING of all things UNDER HEAVEN."

正 言 若 反。

zhèng   *yán*   *ruò*   *fǎn.*

STRAIGHT   SPEECH   SEEM   CONTRARY.

STRAIGHT SPEECH SEEMS CONTRARY.

Chapter 79

和　大　怨，必　有　餘　怨。

hé　*dà*　*yuàn,*　*bì*　*yǒu*　*yú*　*yuàn.*

RECONCILE　GREAT　GRIEVANCE,　MUST　EXIST　MORE　GRIEVANCE.

In RECONCILING GREAT GRIEVANCES, MORE GRIEVANCES MUST REMAIN.

报　怨　以　德，安　可　以　为　善？

bào　*yuàn*　*yǐ*　*dé,*　*ān*　*kě*　*yǐ*　*wéi*　*shàn?*

RESPOND　GRIEVANCE　USE　VIRTUE,　HOW　CAN　ACT　GOOD?

If one RESPONDS to GRIEVANCES USING VIRTUE, HOW CAN one ENACT GOODNESS?

是　以　圣　人　执　左　契，

shì　*yǐ*　*shèng-*　*rén*　*zhí*　*zuǒ*　*qì,*

BE　WHY　SAGACIOUS-　PERSON　HOLD　LEFT　CONTRACT,

This IS WHY the SAGE HOLDS the LEFT half of the CONTRACT,

而　不　责　于　人。

ér　*bù*　*zé*　*yú*　*rén.*

BUT　NOT　DEMAND　OF　PEOPLE.

BUT makes NO DEMANDS OF PEOPLE.

有　德　司　契；无　德　司　彻。

yǒu　*dé*　*sī*　*qì;*　*wú*　*dé*　*sī*　*chè.*

HAVE　VIRTUE　ATTEND　CONTRACT;　NOT　VIRTUE　ATTEND TAX-COLLECTION.

Those who HAVE VIRTUE ATTEND to the CONTRACT; those who do NOT have VIRTUE ATTEND to COLLECTING TAXES.

天　道　无　亲，常　与　善　人。

tiān　*dào*　*wú*　*qīn,*　*cháng*　*yǔ*　*shàn*　*rén.*

HEAVEN　DAO　NOT　INTIMATE,　ALWAYS　WITH　GOOD　PERSON.

The DAO of HEAVEN has NO PREFERENCES, but is ALWAYS WITH the GOOD PERSON.

小　国　寡　民。

xiǎo　*guó*　*guǎ*　*mín.*
SMALL　COUNTRY　FEW　PEOPLE.

The SMALL COUNTRY has FEW PEOPLE.

使　有　什　伯　之　器　而　不　用;

shǐ　*yǒu*　*shí*　*bó*　*zhī*　*qì*　*ér*　*bú*　*yòng;*
CAUSE　EXIST　MANY　HUNDRED　[PART]　WEAPON　BUT　NOT　USE;

It ENSURES that there ARE MANY HUNDREDS of WEAPONS BUT does NOT USE them;

使　民　重　死　而　不　远　徙。

shǐ　*mín*　*zhòng*　*sǐ*　*ér*　*bù*　*yuǎn*　*xǐ.*
CAUSE　PEOPLE　SERIOUSLY　DEATH　AND　NOT　FAR　TRAVEL.

It ENSURES that the PEOPLE take DEATH SERIOUSLY AND do NOT TRAVEL FAR.

虽　有　舟　舆,　无　所　乘　之;

suī　*yǒu*　*zhōu*　*yú,*　*wú*　*suǒ*　*chéng*　*zhī;*
ALTHOUGH　EXIST　BOAT　CHARIOT,　NOT　[PART]　RIDE　THEM;

ALTHOUGH there ARE BOATS and CHARIOTS, NO ONE USES THEM;

虽　有　甲　兵,　无　所　陈　之;

suī　*yǒu*　*jiǎ*　*bīng,*　*wú*　*suǒ*　*chén*　*zhī;*
ALTHOUGH　EXIST　ARMOR　SOLDIER,　NOT　[PART]　DISPLAY　THEM;

ALTHOUGH there ARE ARMOR and SOLDIERS, NO ONE DISPLAYS THEM;

使　民　复　结　绳　而　用　之。

shǐ　*mín*　*fù*　*jié*　*shéng*　*ér*　*yòng*　*zhī.*
CAUSE　PEOPLE　RETURN　TIE　ROPE　AND　USE　THEM.

It ENSURES that the PEOPLE RETURN to TYING ROPES AND USING THEM in lieu of writing.

至　治　之　极。

zhì　zhì　zhī　jí.

ACHIEVE GOVERNMENT [PART] EXTREME.

It ACHIEVES EXCELLENCE IN GOVERNMENT.

甘　其　食;　美　其　服;

gān　qí　shí;　měi　qí　fú;

SWEET ITS FOOD; BEAUTIFUL ITS CLOTHING;

The FOOD is SWEET; the CLOTHING is BEAUTIFUL;

安　其　居;　乐　其　俗。

ān　qí　jū;　lè　qí　sú.

PEACEFUL ITS DWELLING; JOYFUL ITS CUSTOM.

the DWELLINGS are PEACEFUL; the CUSTOMS are JOYFUL.

邻　国　相　望;

lín　guó　xiāng　wàng;

NEIGHBOR COUNTRY MUTUALLY OBSERVE;

NEIGHBORING COUNTRIES MUTUALLY OBSERVE one another;

鸡　犬　之　声　相　闻;

jī　quǎn　zhī　shēng　xiāng　wén;

CHICKEN DOG [PART] SOUND MUTUALLY HEAR;

The SOUNDS of CHICKENS and DOGS are HEARD on BOTH sides;

民　至　老　死,　不　相　往　来。

mín　zhì　lǎo　sǐ,　bù　xiāng　wǎng-　lái.

PEOPLE UNTIL OLD DIE, NOT MUTUALLY GO- COME.

The PEOPLE live UNTIL they DIE of OLD age, but do NOT MUTUALLY COME and GO.

Chapter 81

信　言　不　美；　美　言　不　信。

xìn　yán　bù　měi;　měi　yán　bú　xìn.

BELIEVABLE　WORD　NOT　BEAUTIFUL;　BEAUTIFUL　WORD　NOT　BELIEVABLE.

BELIEVABLE WORDS are NOT BEAUTIFUL; BEAUTIFUL WORDS are NOT BELIEVABLE.

善　者　不　辩；　辩　者　不　善。

shàn　zhě　bú　biàn;　biàn　zhě　bú　shàn.

GOOD　[PART]　NOT　DEBATE;　DEBATE　[PART]　NOT　GOOD.

Those WHO are GOOD do NOT DEBATE; those WHO DEBATE are NOT GOOD.

知　者　不　博；　博　者　不　知。

zhī　zhě　bù　bó;　bó　zhě　bù　zhī.

KNOW　[PART]　NOT　ERUDITE;　ERUDITE　[PART]　NOT　KNOW.

Those WHO KNOW are NOT ERUDITE; those WHO are ERUDITE do NOT KNOW.

圣　人　不　积。

shèng-　rén　bù　jǐ.

SAGACIOUS-　PERSON　NOT　ACCUMULATE.

The SAGE does NOT ACCUMULATE things.

既　以　为　人，　己　愈　有；

jì　yǐ　wéi　rén,　jǐ　yù　yǒu;

SINCE　[PART]　ACT　PEOPLE,　SELF　MORE　HAVE;

SINCE he ACTS for the PEOPLE, he HAS MORE for HIMSELF;

既　以　与　人，　己　愈　多。

jì　yǐ　yǔ　rén,　jǐ　yù　duō.

SINCE　[PART]　GIVE　PEOPLE,　SELF　MORE　GAIN.

SINCE he GIVES to the PEOPLE, he GAINS MORE for HIMSELF.

天　　之　　道，利　　而　　不　　害。

tiān　　zhī　　dào,　　lì　　ér　　bú　　hài.

HEAVEN　[PART]　DAO,　BENEFIT　AND　NOT　HARM.

The DAO OF HEAVEN BENEFITS AND does NOT HARM.

圣　　人　　之　　道，为　　而　　不　　争。

shèng-　　rén　　zhī　　dào,　　wéi　　ér　　bù　　zhēng.

SAGACIOUS-　PERSON　[PART]　DAO,　ACT　BUT　NOT　CONTEND.

The DAO OF THE SAGE ACTS BUT does NOT CONTEND.

Daoism Online

Here is a partial listing of web sites focusing on Daoism. Links are active as of January 1998, and because of the fluid nature of the internet, may change constantly.

To see the traditional characters of the text of the Daodejing, see **Zhongwen.com**. (www.zhongwen.com) Maintained by Rick Harbaugh of Yale University, it contains other classic texts as well as a very useful on-line dictionary to help you look up each character of the text.

Daoism Depot (www.edepot.com/taoism.html) contains lively discussions on Daoism, with Live Chats, links to other related sites, art, a guide to the Chinese characters, and other related subjects (I Ching, the Art of War, etc.). Recommended!

Links Related to the Tao Te Ching (www.teleport.com/~cooler/TAO/tao_related.html) This useful site has the complete text in Chinese, complete translations by various authors (including the first English translation by James Legge) and links to many other related sites.

Taoism Information Page (www.clas.ufl.edu/users/gthursby/taoism/) Another wide-ranging site with links to other sources.

The publisher also maintains a page on new and related sites at the China Books site (www.chinabooks.com)